Surgical Approach to Incontinence

Guest Editor

ROGER R. DMOCHOWSKI, MD

UROLOGIC CLINICS OF NORTH AMERICA

www.urologic.theclinics.com

February 2011 • Volume 38 • Number 1

SAUNDERS an imprint of ELSEVIER, Inc.

W.B. SAUNDERS COMPANY
A Division of Elsevier Inc.

1600 John F. Kennedy Blvd. • Suite 1800 • Philadelphia, PA 19103-2899

http://www.theclinics.com

UROLOGIC CLINICS OF NORTH AMERICA Volume 38, Number 1
February 2011 ISSN 0094-0143, ISBN-13: 978-1-4557-0708-9

Editor: Stephanie Donley

Urologic Clinics of North America (ISSN 0094-0143) is published quarterly by Elsevier Inc., 360 Park Avenue South, New York, NY 10010-1710. Months of issue are February, May, August, and November. Business and Editorial Offices: 1600 John F. Kennedy Blvd., Suite 1800, Philadelphia, PA 19103-2899. Periodicals postage paid at New York, NY and additional mailing offices. Subscription prices are $311.00 per year (US individuals), $519.00 per year (US institutions), $363.00 per year (Canadian individuals), $636.00 per year (Canadian institutions), $451.00 per year (foreign individuals), and $636.00 per year (foreign institutions). Foreign air speed delivery is included in all *Clinics* subscription prices. All prices are subject to change without notice. **POSTMASTER:** Send address changes to *Urologic Clinics of North America*, Elsevier Health Sciences Division, Subscription Customer Service, 3251 Riverport Lane, Maryland Heights, MO 63043. Customer Service: 1-800-654-2452 (US). From outside the United States, call 1-314-447-8871. Fax: 1-314-447-8029. E-mail: JournalsCustomerServiceusa@elsevier.com (for print support) and JournalsOnlineSupport-usa@elsevier.com (for online support).

Reprints. For copies of 100 or more, of articles in this publication, please contact the Commercial Reprints Department, Elsevier Inc., 360 Park Avenue South, New York, New York 10010-1710. Tel.: 212-633-3813; Fax: 212-462-1935; E-mail: reprints@elsevier.com.

Urologic Clinics of North America is covered in MEDLINE/PubMed (*Index Medicus*), *Excerpta Medica, Current Contents/Clinical Medicine, Science Citation Index,* and *ISI/BIOMED.*

Printed and bound by CPI Group (UK) Ltd, Croydon, CR0 4YY
Transferred to Digital Print 2011

Contributors

GUEST EDITOR

ROGER R. DMOCHOWSKI, MD, FACS
Professor of Urologic Surgery; Director Pelvic
Reconstructive Surgery Fellowship, Vanderbilt
University Medical Center; Executive Physician
for Safety, Department of Urology, Vanderbilt
University Hospital, Nashville, Tennessee

AUTHORS

†RODNEY A. APPELL, MD, FACS
Professor of Urology and Gynecology and
Chief, Division of Voiding Dysfunction and
Female Urology, Department of Urology,
Baylor College of Medicine; F. Brantley Scott
Chair in Urology, St. Luke's Episcopal Hospital,
Houston, Texas

JERRY G. BLAIVAS, MD
Clinical Professor of Urology, Weil Cornell
Medical School; Adjunct Professor of
Urology, SUNY Downstate Medical School,
New York, New York

R. DUANE CESPEDES, MD
Director of Female Urology and Urodynamics,
Department of Urology, Wilford Hall Medical
Center, Lackland Air Force Base, Texas

DAVID C. CHAIKIN, MD
Clinical Assistant Professor of Urology,
Department of Urology, Sanford Weil
Medical Center of Cornell University,
New York, New York; Vice President,
Garden State Urology, Attending Urologist
Morristown Memorial Hospital,
Morristown, New Jersey

EMILY E. COLE, MD
Assistant Professor of Urology, Department
of Urology, Uniformed Services, University
of the Health Sciences; Staff Urologist, Naval
Medical Center, San Diego, California

ROGER R. DMOCHOWSKI, MD, FACS
Professor of Urologic Surgery; Director Pelvic
Reconstructive Surgery Fellowship, Vanderbilt
University Medical Center; Executive Physician
for Safety, Department of Urology, Vanderbilt
University Hospital, Nashville, Tennessee

HOWARD B. GOLDMAN, MD
Associate Professor of Urology, Center for
Female Pelvic Medicine and Reconstructive
Surgery, Glickman Urologic and Kidney
Institute, The Cleveland Clinic Lerner
College of Medicine, Case Western
Reserve University, Cleveland, Ohio

MICKEY M. KARRAM, MD
Director of Urogynecology & Reconstructive
Pelvic Surgery, The Christ Hospital;
Clinical Professor of Obstetrics and
Gynecology, University of Cincinnati;
Clinical Professor of Urology, Department
of Surgery, University of Cincinnati,
Cincinnati, Ohio

STEVEN D. KLEEMAN, MD
Director, Division of Urogynecology,
Department of Obstetrics & Gynecology,
Good Samaritan Hospital; Director,
Female Pelvic Medicine and Reconstructive
Surgery Fellowship Program, Good
Samaritan Hospital, Cincinnati, Ohio

†Deceased.

PATRICK B. LEU, MD
Clinical Assistant Professor of Surgery,
Urology, University of Nebraska Medical
Center, Omaha, Nebraska

VICTOR W. NITTI, MD
Professor and Vice Chairman, Department
of Urology, New York University, Langone
Medical Center, New York, New York

ANDREW C. PETERSON, MD
Associate Professor of Urologic Surgery,
Division of Urology, Duke University Medical
Center, Durham, North Carolina

NIRIT ROSENBLUM, MD
Assistant Professor of Urology, Female Pelvic
Medicine & Voiding Dysfunction, New York
University, Langone Medical Center,
New York, New York

HARRIETTE M. SCARPERO, MD
Associated Urologists, Department
of Urologic Surgery, Vanderbilt Continence
Center, Vanderbilt University Medical Center,
Nashville, Tennessee

JOSEPH A. SMITH Jr, MD
Professor and Chairman, Department
of Urologic Surgery, Vanderbilt University
Medical Center, Nashville, Tennessee

GEORGE D. WEBSTER, MB, FRCS
Department of Urologic Surgery, Duke
University Medical Center, Durham,
North California

J. CHRISTIAN WINTERS, MD
Department of Urology, Ochsner Clinic
Foundation, New Orleans, Louisiana

Contents

bulbourethral sling and treatment of neurogenic bladder with the prostatic urethral sling. Men with mild-to-moderate intrinsic sphincteric dysfunction after prostatectomy seem to be appropriate candidates for the bone-anchored bulbourethral sling, and the prostatic urethral sling may be an acceptable substitute in patients with neurogenic bladder with intrinsic sphincteric dysfunction.

Since its introduction in 1973, the artificial urinary sphincter (AUS) has become widely accepted therapy, particularly for male incontinence. In this article, the authors review their experience with more than 600 artificial urinary sphincter (AUS) devices and discuss practical points concerning surgery and revisions. Their routine surgical approach as a means of reporting on technical lessons learned is also described.

GOAL STATEMENT

The goal of *Urologic Clinics of North America* is to keep practicing urologists and urology residents up to date with current clinical practice in urology by providing timely articles reviewing the state of the art in patient care.

ACCREDITATION

The *Urologic Clinics of North America* is planned and implemented in accordance with the Essential Areas and Policies of the Accreditation Council for Continuing Medical Education (ACCME) through the joint sponsorship of the University of Virginia School of Medicine and Elsevier. The University of Virginia School of Medicine is accredited by the ACCME to provide continuing medical education for physicians.

The University of Virginia School of Medicine designates this educational activity for a maximum of 15 *AMA PRA Category 1 Credits*™ for each issue, 60 credits per year. Physicians should only claim credit commensurate with the extent of their participation in the activity.

The American Medical Association has determined that physicians not licensed in the US who participate in this CME activity are eligible for a maximum of 15 *AMA PRA Category 1 Credits*™ for each issue, 60 credits per year.

Credit can be earned by reading the text material, taking the CME examination online at http://www.theclinics.com/home/cme, and completing the evaluation. After taking the test, you will be required to review any and all incorrect answers. Following completion of the test and evaluation, your credit will be awarded and you may print your certificate.

FACULTY DISCLOSURE/CONFLICT OF INTEREST

The University of Virginia School of Medicine, as an ACCME accredited provider, endorses and strives to comply with the Accreditation Council for Continuing Medical Education (ACCME) Standards of Commercial Support, Commonwealth of Virginia statutes, University of Virginia policies and procedures, and associated federal and private regulations and guidelines on the need for disclosure and monitoring of proprietary and financial interests that may affect the scientific integrity and balance of content delivered in continuing medical education activities under our auspices.

The University of Virginia School of Medicine requires that all CME activities accredited through this institution be developed independently and be scientifically rigorous, balanced and objective in the presentation/discussion of its content, theories and practices.

All authors/editors participating in an accredited CME activity are expected to disclose to the readers relevant financial relationships with commercial entities occurring within the past 12 months (such as grants or research support, employee, consultant, stock holder, member of speakers bureau, etc.). The University of Virginia School of Medicine will employ appropriate mechanisms to resolve potential conflicts of interest to maintain the standards of fair and balanced education to the reader. Questions about specific strategies can be directed to the Office of Continuing Medical Education, University of Virginia School of Medicine, Charlottesville, Virginia.

The faculty and staff of the University of Virginia Office of Continuing Medical Education have no financial affiliations to disclose.

The authors/editors listed below have identified no professional or financial affiliations for themselves or their spouse/partner:
R. Duane Cespedes, MD; Howard B. Goldman, MD; Kerry Holland, (Acquisitions Editor); Steven D. Kleeman, MD; Patrick B. Leu, MD; Andrew C. Peterson, MD; Nirit Rosenblum, MD; and Joseph A. Smith Jr, MD.

The authors/editors listed below identified the following professional or financial affiliations for themselves or their spouse/partner:
Jerry G. Blaivas, MD is a consultant for Pfizer and Merck, and owns stock in HDH and Endogun.
David C. Chaikin, MD is a consultant for Warner Chilcott, and is on the Speakers' Bureau for Pfizer.
Emily E. Cole, MD is a consultant for Pfizer.
Roger R. Dmochowski, MD (Guest Editor) is a consultant for Pfizer, Astellas, Alergan, and Johnson & Johnson.
Mickey M. Karram, MD is a consultant and is on the Speakers' Bureau for Astellas Pharma, EWH & U, and AMS.
Victor W. Nitti, MD is a consultant and is on the Advisory Committee/Board for Allergan, Astellas, Coloplast, Ethicon, Serenity Pharmaceuticals, and Uroplasty; is an industry funded research/investigator for Allergan and Coloplast; is a consultant for American Medical Systems; and is on the Advisory Committee/Board for Medtronic and Pfizer.
Harriette M. Scarpero, MD is on the Advisory Committee/Board for American Medical Systems, and is an industry funded research/investigator for Pfizer, Inc.
William Steers, MD (Test Author) is employed by the American Urologic Association, is a reviewer and consultant for NIH, and is an investigator for Allergan.
George D. Webster, MB, FRCS is a consultant for American Medical Systems, Inc, and is a lecturer for Life Tech, Inc.
J. Christian Winters, MD is a consultant for Astellas, Inc. and Pfizer, Inc.

Disclosure of Discussion of Non-FDA Approved Uses for Pharmaceutical Products and/or Medical Devices.
The University of Virginia School of Medicine, as an ACCME provider, requires that all faculty presenters identify and disclose any off-label uses for pharmaceutical and medical device products. The University of Virginia School of Medicine recommends that each physician fully review all the available data on new products or procedures prior to clinical use.

TO ENROLL

To enroll in the Urologic Clinics of North America Continuing Medical Education program, call customer service at 1-800-654-2452 or visit us online at www.theclinics.com/home/cme. The CME program is available to subscribers for an additional fee of $207.00.

Urologic Clinics of North America

THE CLINICS ARE NOW AVAILABLE ONLINE!

Access your subscription at:
www.theclinics.com

Preface

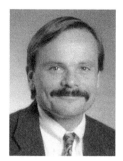

Roger R. Dmochowski, MD
Guest Editor

This Atlas represents a reprinting of a previously published document which summarized advancements in incontinence surgery. As will be noted from the table of contents several of the included chapters dealt with topics that have undergone substantial technical change and innovation since the first publication. The authors represent a distinguished group of leaders in the field of incontinence surgery. They have summarized their approaches and procedural nuances to a variety of interventions for incontinence in women (including prolapse and stress incontinence) and male incontinence. Also included is an update on reconstructive pelvic surgery in female patients with invasive bladder cancer.

As noted in the preface of the first edition of this book, "State of the Art" procedures are relevant only until changes in technology and/or improved understanding of pathophysiology mandate alterations either in procedure or strategy/indications for procedures. Specifically, the interested reader will note there has been further evolution in types of midurethral slings available and insertion techniques associated with these varied procedures.

Additionally, the advent of the use of various mesh procedures for prolapse repair has led to substantial technological change for some approaches to the management of pelvic prolapse. However, the ultimate impact on outcomes of these procedural types remains, as yet, uncertain.

What is clear is that with the aging demographics of our population, incontinence procedures will continue to be an important aspect of the panoply of treatments for lower urinary tract dysfunction. It is reasonable to assume that these procedures will continue to evolve and that the interested surgeon and practitioner remain abreast of current literature and technological advancements related to this field.

Roger R. Dmochowski, MD
Department of Urologic Surgery
Vanderbilt University Medical Center
Room A-1302, Medical Center North
Nashville, TN 37232-2765, USA

E-mail address:
Roger.dmochowski@vanderbilt.edu

Urol Clin N Am 38 (2011) xi
doi:10.1016/j.ucl.2011.01.001

Urethral and Bladder Injections for Incontinence Including Botox

Rodney A. Appell, MD[a,b,†]

KEYWORDS

- Endoscopic injection therapy • Periurethral bulking agents
- Botox injections

Stress urinary incontinence (SUI) and urge incontinence (UI) are increasingly significant health concerns for millions of women. Approximately 180,000 surgical procedures are performed for genuine SUI alone. The lack of a single, reproducible, permanent, and minimal-risk procedure has led to the development of several minimally invasive options that provide the hope of reasonable efficacy and minimal morbidity. Reimbursement trends have placed an emphasis on interventions that require minimal hospitalization or that can be performed in the ambulatory office without the use of general or regional anesthesia and attendant recuperative facilities.

Injection therapy has been used sparingly for the management of SUI for nearly 2 decades, but has been limited by durability and antigenicity issues associated with bovine collagen. Food and Drug Administration (FDA) approval of carbon particulate technology (Durasphere) has provided another option for bulking, but this treatment is limited by difficulty with injection (because carrier extrusion can result in injection-needle obstruction).

Because of these concerns, many physicians would use Durasphere only in the controlled setting of the operative suite, detracting from the financial benefit associated with in-office bulking therapy. This issue was addressed by the manufacturer, and an improved formulation (Durasphere EXP) was introduced after FDA approval was given in October 2003; injection of this treatment is as easy as injection of collagen. The use of bulking therapy had been less than optimal; however, the advent of several new bulking agents (each with unique tissue-interaction characteristics, the promise of greater durability, fewer injection sessions, and no antigenicity) promises to alter the role of bulking therapy in the overall management schema for SUI. Selection of patients seems to be crucial to the outcome of the intraurethral injection of bulking agents. The ideal candidate for this procedure has good anatomic support; a compliant, stable bladder; and a malfunctioning urethra as evidenced by a low leak point pressure. Other patients who may benefit from the procedure are patients with high leak point pressure

A version of this article was previously published in the *Atlas of the Urologic Clinics of North America* 12:2.
[a] Division of Voiding Dysfunction and Female Urology, Department of Urology, Baylor College of Medicine, 6560 Fannin Street, Suite #2100, Houston, TX 77030, USA
[b] St. Luke's Episcopal Hospital, 6720 Bertner Street, Houston, TX 77030, USA
[†]Deceased.

and minimal hypermobility and elderly women with bladder base mobility who are less active and are a poor surgical risk for other interventions.

Investigation continues into the use of different types of procedures for the surgical management of UI. These procedures lend themselves to the ambulatory or office setting and mimic the efficacy and safety profiles of currently available procedures (such as sacral nerve neuromodulation).

INJECTABLE AGENTS FOR TREATING SUI

The successful use of periurethral bulking agents is dependent on several factors, such as the composition of the material, the facility of agent use (ease of preparation and implantation), and a receptive host environment (optimized hormonal environment, integrity of urethral anatomic components, intact periurethral fascia). Three categories of materials have been investigated for periurethral bulking: human (autologous or allograft), xenograft, and synthetic.

The optimal attributes for bulking materials are biocompatibility, minimal or no immunogenicity (hypoallergenic), and integrity of the material formulation (there should be little or no separation of agent subcomponents [carrier and particulate solid]). Rheologic (deformation within tissue) characteristics of the agent should be affected positively by adequate material viscosity, surface tension, and tissue response (wound healing). These attributes for any specific agent should be reproducible. Tissue-response characteristics should demonstrate minimal fibrotic ingrowth and little extracapsular inflammatory response (if encapsulation occurs). Agent volume after injection should be retained with minimal resorption. The most ideal scenario for any soft tissue-bulking agent is a single injection with permanent tissue residence of the agent (and partial or total incorporation into the host tissues); however, available agents do not ideally fulfill these criteria because of isolated or combined agent and host factors (eg, lack of resorption, agent admixture separation).

The goal of endoscopic injection therapy for SUI is to provide a minimally invasive, effective, and safe alternative to open surgery. Although the technique has been available for decades, the ideal injectable material has yet to be developed. In addition to being biocompatible, nonantigenic, noninfectious, and noncarcinogenic, the material must demonstrate anatomic integrity. This requirement implies that the material conserves its volume over time. Although bovine collagen is safe for use as injection treatment for SUI, it lacks this anatomic integrity. This fact reduces the ability of collagen to be cost effective.[7] A significant

volume is required at each injection session, and multiple injection sessions are the rule, reducing cost effectiveness and resulting in patient inconvenience and patient dissatisfaction with collagen or injectable therapy in general. Information on collagen has been well documented.[8]

Treatment with Durasphere pyrolytic carbon-coated zirconium oxide beads was approved by the FDA in 1999. The beads are suspended in a water-soluble β-glucan vehicle. The randomized, multicenter, double-blind study that was accepted by the FDA showed that collagen and Durasphere had similar outcomes and that the original Durasphere had a slight benefit. Durasphere is more viscous than collagen, and as mentioned earlier, its injection was more technically demanding than that with collagen (although injection has become easier with the introduction of Durasphere-EXP). Renewed concern has been expressed about material migration after injection. Microcrystalline components of the bulking agent should be composed of uniform spheroidal particles sized greater than 80 μm (the approximate size required to avoid migration as determined in studies involving polytetrafluoroethylene [Teflon]). Migration is influenced by the ability of host macrophages to phagocytize particles, and smaller particle sizes have been shown to migrate to distant locations with Teflon injection. Direct embolization of material is caused by high-pressure injection, resulting in material displacement into vascular or lymphatic spaces. Injection technique should rely on larger-sized particles that are administered with low-pressure injection instrumentation.[1] This requirement should not be a problem with Durasphere-EXP, as its particles range in size from 95 to 200 μm, whereas the particles in the original Durasphere are significantly smaller (200–550 μm); however, the Durasphere-EXP's smallest particles are still greater in size than the 80 μm needed for safety.

Agents in Development

Synthetic calcium hydoxylapatite is identical to the material found in human teeth and bones. The agent is composed of hydroxylapatite spheres (which are uniform in shape, smooth, and 75–125 μm in size) in an aqueous gel composed of sodium carboxylmethylcellulose (Coaptite). Plain film radiography or ultrasonography may be used localize this material and can be useful adjuncts to assessing implantation. The first FDA-approved indication for this material has been obtained, specifically for soft tissue marking as an adjunct to radiographic focusing for radiotherapeutics. Agent injection is performed with a small bore

(21-gauge needle) and standard cystoscopic instruments. An ongoing, large-scale North American pivotal trial is accruing more than 250 women. Twenty-one women have received Coaptite, 18 women received collagen, and the subjects have been followed for 1 year since last injection.[2] The average number of injections was 2.0 for Coaptite and 2.3 for collagen. The total volume injected was 3.7 mL for Coaptite and 7.4 mL for collagen. Eighty-six percent of Coaptite recipients improved by at least one Stamey grade, 67% improved by two grades, and 38% were completely continent, whereas among collagen recipients, the respective percentages were 66%, 55%, and 44%. Overall pad weight reduction in a 1-hour stress pad test was at least 75% in 77% of Coaptite recipients but in only 55% of collagen recipients; reduction of 90% or greater occurred in 46% of Coaptite recipients and 33% of collagen recipients. No prolonged retention, urgency, or periurethral erosion or abscess was seen in either group. This agent has similar injection characteristics to collagen and seems to require a lower injected volume for a somewhat more durable effect.

Another biologic agent, Zuidex, consists of dextranomer microspheres in a cross-linked hyaluronic acid (HA) vehicle. HA is a water-insoluble, complex glycosaminoglycan that is composed of disaccharide units, which form molecules of 23 million molecular weight, and is dissolved in normal saline for urethral bulking purposes. This composite gel has significant elasticity and high viscosity. These biologic characteristics have led to the use of hylan gels for soft tissue bulking purposes. It is completely biodegradable and nonimmunogenic. HA functions as the transport compound and is resorbed within 2 weeks after injection. The dextranomer microspheres function as the bulking agent, are 80 to 200 μm in size, do not show fragility with insertion, and remain in the injection site for about 4 years. Injection is performed using standard cystoscopic equipment with minimal injection pressure. An ongoing clinical trial in the United States is evaluating this agent for treating SUI. The technique for HA injection does not require endoscopy. A small device is placed into the urethra, and the needles direct the injected material in 1-mL aliquots at the midurethra. Substantive data have shown the efficacy and safety of this agent, allowing FDA approval for use in treating vesicoureteral reflux and pediatric incontinence. The site for incontinence injections is the bladder neck, as had been the convention for the treatment of SUI until this new trial of HA in women with SUI.

Results of dextranomer injection for pediatric incontinence showed no associated adverse events and substantial improvement 12 months after injection.[3] Sixteen patients (with a variety of underlying causes for their incontinence) underwent a mean of 2.3 injections (mean volume, 2.8 mL) and subsequent annual follow-up. According to 1-hour pad tests and diary data, 75% of patients improved at 6 months, and 50% improved at 12 months. Follow-up at 2 years indicated relative stability of incontinence parameters, as compared with 1-year data. No local injection-site complications or immunologic sequelae resulted. Similar durability and safety findings have been identified with this material when used for the reflux indication.

Synthetic agents pose a potential benefit as bulking agents because of their stability (nonbiodegradability). Silicone is a hydrogel suspension that has polyvinylpyrrolidone (povidone) as the carrier (which also acts as a lubricant for the injection system) and solid polydimethylsiloxane elastomer (vulcanized silicone) as the bulking agent. The elastomer is a particulate of varying shapes and conformal configurations. Particle size is markedly variable; 25% of particles are less than 50 μm in size, and some particles are greater than 400 μm in size. Silicone delivery requires high-pressure administration, but with newer equipment allows easier delivery of this material. Although the use of silicone is well established in Europe, concerns regarding silicone stimulation of the immunologic response have limited evaluation of this agent in the United States. A clinical trial evaluating the use of Macroplastique (a type of silicone) as a bulking agent is in progress in North America. A Scandinavian report followed 22 women for 2 years after receiving a silicone injection.[4] Subjective and objective criteria showed stability and persistent benefit. Overall pad test data showed dramatic reduction (mean pretreatment level, 147 g; mean post-treatment level, 9 g). No long-term local or systemic complications were noted.

Ethylene vinyl alcohol copolymer suspended in dimethyl sulfoxide or Uryx solution is being evaluated as an embolic agent and a bulking agent. On injection and exposure to solution (blood or extracellular space) at physiologic temperatures, the dimethyl sulfoxide diffuses from the co-polymer and causes the ethylene vinyl alcohol to precipitate into a complex spongiform mass. This phase change requires diligent separation of the agent and body-temperature fluids until implantation occurs. Early experience with this agent suggested that optimal results can be obtained with injection in a slightly more distal urethral location within the urethra (approximately 1.5 cm distal to the bladder neck); with a slower rate of injection (at least 30 s/mL/injection site); and without the need to observe visual coaptation at the completion of injection, as the volume injected is limited to 2.5 mL on each side of the urethra. Using these end-point criteria, results have been good. With this material, injection is done with this set volume rather than with an end point of coaptation of the urethra or bladder neck at the time of injection. A large-scale North American trial is in progress. The trial incorporated 237 women with genuine SUI and used a prospective, randomized (Uryx-to-bovine collagen ratio, 2:1) schema.[5] Treated patients were for 1 year after last injection. At 6 months, 40 Uryx recipients and 23 collagen recipients have been evaluated (at 12 months, 21 and 13 subjects, respectively, had been evaluated). The mean total volume of material required for injection was lower for Uryx (4.4 mL) than for collagen (6.9 mL). At 6 months, 63% of Uryx recipients are dry (no incontinent episodes), compared with 48% of collagen recipients. At 12 months, 74% of Uryx recipients were dry, compared with 40% of collagen recipients. Rates of postimplantation urgency and dysuria were similar between the two arms. This result suggests that, unlike collagen, Uryx maintains a durability of response that has not been noted with biologic agents and may be the first synthetic material to do this without substantive complication issues.

A requirement for FDA trials with these agents is active comparison with bovine collagen. No head-to-head data exist between these evolving agents for treating genuine SUI; however, one trial has compared Macroplastique with dextranomer and HA for the treatment of ureteral reflux in children.[6]

INJECTABLE AGENTS FOR TREATING UI

Attempts at this treatment modality first were reported in 1969 with subtrigonal injections of 6% (aqueous) phenol.[9] Injection of phenol causes neurolysis of terminal pelvic nerve branches as they enter the trigone. Approximately 10 to 20 mL of the material is injected through a cystoscope in the submucosal level, bilaterally halfway between the bladder neck and each ureteral orifice. The procedure requires general or regional anesthesia. This treatment modality has yielded mixed results. Some investigators reported success rates as high as 82% to 90%,[10,11] whereas others reported poor success rates of less than 20%.[12] Some studies attempted to identify subcategories of patients who were most likely to benefit from this procedure. Blackford and colleagues[10] reported a success rate of 82% in women with multiple sclerosis older than 55 and less than 14% in women younger than 55. To improve patient selection, Madjar and colleagues[13] used a transvaginal bupivacaine injection (0.25%) on the assumption that patients who respond to the local anesthetic

later will respond to the subtrigonal phenol injection. In their study, 23 of 42 patients (54.7%) responded to the bupivacaine injection. Of the patients who responded to the phenol injections, 26% had symptomatic relief that lasted more than 3 months. In most cases, relief of symptoms was temporary and lasted from a few weeks to several months. Severe complications, such as vesicovaginal fistulas, excoriation of the vaginal wall, and the need for urinary diversion, were reported in 25% to 40% of patients in two series.[11,14] In these patients, the phenol was mixed in a nonaqueous, glycerol solution, which retained the phenol in the perivesical fat for a longer period of time. Because of the high complication rate, many physicians consider previous pelvic surgery or pelvic irradiation to be contraindications for this treatment.

Botulinum toxin (Botox) has proved to be a safe and effective therapy for a variety of somatic and autonomic motor disorders and seems to have some clinical efficacy in the treatment of detrusor-external sphincter-dyssynergia (DESD), pelvic floor spasticity, and overacitve bladder. The toxin acts by inhibiting acetylcholine release at the presynaptic cholinergic junction. Clinically, Botox has been used to treat patients with spinal cord injury, DESD,[15] and neurogenic detrusor overactivity,[16] resulting in a significant reduction in maximum detrusor voiding pressure. A long-term study of detrusor overactivity in 87 patients reported that the clinical response lasted only 4 to 14 months, but no adverse events occurred.[17] Although treatment with botulinum toxin is safe, the maintenance of clinical results requires repeated transcystoscopic injections. This agent is expensive and is not reimbursed by health insurance companies for use in urologic injection, as it is not FDA approved to treat any indication involving the urinary tract. Costs can be reduced by doing the procedure under local anesthesia in an office setting.

A TECHNIQUE FOR BOTOX INJECTION INTO THE BLADDER UNDER LOCAL ANESTHESIA

I anesthetize the urethra with 2% lidocaine jelly, empty the bladder, instill 50 mL of 1% plain lidocaine solution, and let the solution remain for 10 minutes before placing the cystoscope and beginning the injections. I inject 100 U in 0.5-mL (5 U of Botox) aliquots across the back of the trigone (20 small injections in total). I inject another 100 U in radial fashion from the trigone, up the posterior wall, and toward the dome of the bladder. In this portion, five injections are done in each of four radial positions (**Fig. 1**). Other techniques for the injection, such as the concentration of Botox, have not been reported to be more effective than another.

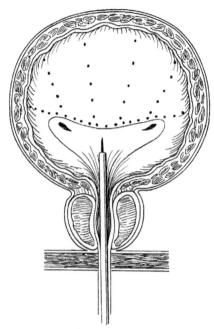

Fig. 1. Technique for bladder chemodenervation with Botox.

The technique also has been used in patients with idiopathic overactive bladder. In a pilot study, Radziszewski and colleagues[18] reported favorably on intravesical Botox A injection to treat overactive bladder and functional outlet obstruction. After intravesical or sphincteric injections, there was resolution of incontinence and improved voiding efficiency, respectively, but for only a short duration.

Chemical denervation of the external sphincter begins within 2 to 3 days and is reversed within 3 to 6 months as terminal nerve sprouting occurs.[19] Dykstra and Sidi published the only double-blind, placebo-controlled study of Botox A. In the Botox recipients, the urethral pressure decreased an average of 25-cm H_2O, postvoid residual decreased an average of 125 mL, and detrusor pressure during voiding decreased an average of 30-cm H_2O. In placebo (normal saline injection) recipients, these factors were unchanged. A study by Phelan and colleagues[20] confirmed these findings: At between 3 and 16 months after injection, the reduction in voiding pressures was 38%.

SUMMARY

Injectable treatment for SUI and UI can be effective and safe; however, the durability of the positive result remains a primary concern when implementing these minimally invasive techniques. With time and further research improvements, the use of injectable agents for treating SUI is inevitable.

Chemical denervation for detrusor and sphincter overactivity is in its infancy. The dose and volume injected seem to have important roles in inducing results and probably relate to possible systemic toxicity. Targets for future chemical denervation go beyond DESD and detrusor motor overactivity; involve various forms of bladder neck obstruction, including benign prostatic hyperplasia; and perhaps will move into the sensory and urgency realms, which might include interstitial cystitis.

REFERENCES

1. Ritts RE. Particle migration after transurethral injection of carbon coated beads. J Urol 2002;167:1804–5.
2. Dmochowski R, Appell RA, Klimberg I, et al. Initial clinical results from coaptite injection for stress urinary incontinence, comparative clinical study. In: Program of the International Continence Society. Heidelberg: 2002.
3. Caione P, Capozza N. Endoscopic treatment of urinary incontinence in pediatric patients: 2 year experience with dextranomer/hyaluronic acid. J Urol 2002;168:1868–71.
4. Peeker R, Edlund C, Wennberg AL, et al. The treatment of sphincter incontinence with periurethral silicone implant (Macroplastique). Scand J Urol Nephrol 2002;36:194–8.
5. Dmochowski RR, Herschorn S, Corcos J, et al. Multicenter randomized controlled study to evaluate Uryx urethral bulking agent in treating female stress urinary incontinence. J Urol 2002;167: LB-10 (A).
6. Aboutaleb H, Bolduc S, Upadhyay J, et al. Subureteral polydimethylsiloxane injection versus extravesical reimplantation for primary low grade vesicoureteral reflux in children: a comparative study. J Urol 2002;169:313–6.
7. Culligan PJ, Rackley R, Koduri S, et al. Is it safe to reuse a syringe of glutaraldehyde cross-linked collagen? A microbiological study. J Urol 2000;164:1275–6.
8. Kershen RT, Dmochowski RR, Appell RA. Beyond collagen: injectable therapies for the treatment of female stress urinary incontinence in the new millennium. Urol Clin N Am 2002;29:559–74.
9. Susset JG, Pinheiro J, Otton P, et al. Selective phenolization and neurotomy in the treatment of neurogenic bladder dusfunction due to an incomplete central lesion. J Urol Nephrol (Paris) 1969;75(12 Suppl):502.
10. Blackford HN, Murray K, Stephenson TP, et al. Results of transvesical infiltration of the pelvic plexuses with phenol in 116 patients. Br J Urol 1984;56:647–9.
11. Harris RG, Constantinou CE, Stamey TA. Extravesical subtrigonal injection of 50% ethanol for detrusor instability. J Urol 1988;140:116.
12. Ramsey IN, Clancy S, Hilton P. Subtrigonal phenol injections in the treatment of idiopathic detrusor

instability in the female—a long-term urodynamic follow-up. Br J Urol 1992;69:363–5.

13. Madjar S, Smith ND, Balzarro M, et al. Bupivacaine injections prior to subtrigonal phenolization: preliminary results. In: Proceedings of the 22nd Annual Meeting of the Society for Urodynamics and Female Urology. Anaheim (CA); 2001.

14. Bennani S. Evaluation of sub-trigonal injections in the treatment of the hyperactive bladder. Ann Urol 1994;28:13–9.

15. Petit H, Wiart E, Gaujard E, et al. Bulinum A toxin treatment for detrosr-sphincter-dyssynergia in spinal cord disease. Spinal Cord 1998;36:91–4.

16. Schurch B, Stohrer M, Kramer, et al. Botulinum-A toxin for treating detrusor hyper-reflexia in spinal cord injured patients: a new alternative to anticholinergic drugs? Preliminary results. J Urol 2000;164:692–7.

17. Schurch B, Stohrer M, Kramer G, et al. Botulinum toxin A to treat detrusor hyper-reflexia in spinal cord injured patients. Neurourol Urodyn 2001;20:521–2.

18. Radziszewski P, Dobronski P, Borkowski A. Treatment of the non-neurogenic storage and voiding disorders with the chemical denervation caused by botulinum toxin A: a pilot study. Neuroruol Urodyn 2001;20:410–2.

19. de Paiva A, Meunier FA, Molgo J, et al. Functional repair of motor endplates after botulinum neurotoxin type A poisoning: biphasic switch of synaptic activity between nerve sprouts and their parent terminals. Proc Natl Acad Sci USA 1999;96:3200–5.

20. Phelan MW, Franks M, Smogyi GT, et al. Botulinum toxin urethral sphincter injection to restore bladder emptying in men and women with voiding dysfunction. J Urol 2001;165:1107–10.

Pubovaginal Fascial Sling for the Treatment of all Types of Stress Urinary Incontinence: Surgical Technique and Long-term Outcome

Jerry G. Blaivas, MD[a], David C. Chaikin, MD[a,b],*

KEYWORDS

- Burch colposuspension pubovaginal sling
- Autologous rectus fascial slilng
- Simplified urinary incontinence outcome score (SUIOS)

A plethora of surgical techniques has been devised for the treatment of stress urinary incontinence, but over the past decade, two approaches have emerged as the gold standards—the Burch colposuspension and the pubovaginal sling. Historically, use of the pubovaginal sling had been reserved for women with complicated, severe, or recurrent sphincteric incontinence, but has been advocated for almost all types of sphincteric incontinence (simple and complicated). Fueled by a stampede of commercial innovations in sling materials, allograft and synthetic slings have become the most commonly used techniques for treating sphincteric incontinence in women. There is little doubt that some kind of allograft or synthetic sling will replace the autologous fascial sling as the gold-standard treatment. This article provides an update on the surgical technique and long-term outcome of the full-length autologous rectus fascial sling in the treatment of women with sphincteric incontinence.

OPERATIVE TECHNIQUE

The procedure is performed in the dorsal lithotomy position. For most patients, a short (6–8 cm) transverse incision is made just above the pubis below the pubic hairline (**Fig. 1**). In obese patients, a larger incision may be necessary. The incision is carried down to the surface of the rectus fascia, which is dissected free of subcutaneous tissue. Two parallel horizontal incisions are made 2 cm apart in the midline of the rectus fascia about 2 cm above the pubis (**Fig. 2**). Using Mayo scissors, the incisions are extended superolaterally toward the iliac crest following the direction of the fascial fibers. The wound edges are retracted laterally on either side to permit a sling of about 16 cm to be obtained. The undersurface of the fascia is freed from muscle and scar, and each end of the fascia is secured with a 2:0 permanent monofilament suture using a running horizontal mattress placed at right angles to the direction of the fascial fibers (**Fig. 3**). The

A version of this article was previously published in the *Atlas of the Urologic Clinics of North America* 12:2.

[a] Department of Urology, Weil Cornell Medical School, 445 East 77th Street, New York, NY 10075, USA
[b] Morristown Memorial Hospital, 100 Madison Avenue, Morristown, NJ 07962, USA
* Corresponding author. Department of Urology, Weil Cornell Medical School, 445 East 77th Street, New York, NY 10075.
E-mail address: DChaikin@gsunj.com

Urol Clin N Am 38 (2011) 7–15
doi:10.1016/j.ucl.2010.12.002

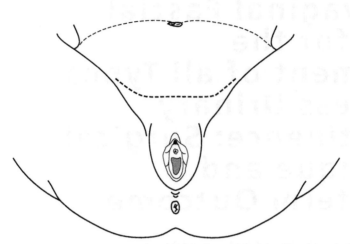

Fig. 1. Abdominal incision. For most patients, a short (6–8 cm) transverse incision is made just above the pubis below the pubic hairline. In obese patients, a larger incision may be necessary.

fascial strip is excised (**Fig. 4**) and placed in a basin of saline. The wound is packed temporarily with saline-soaked sponges, and attention is turned to the vagina.

A weighted vaginal retractor is placed in the vagina, and a Foley catheter is inserted into the urethra. The labia are retracted with sutures. The vesical neck is identified by placing gentle traction on the Foley catheter and palpating the balloon, and a gently curved horizontal incision is made in the anterior vaginal wall. The apex of the curve is over the vesical neck and about 2 cm proximal to the palpable distal edge of the balloon (**Fig. 5**). This incision should be made superficial to the pubocervical fascia. To accomplish this task, an Allis clamp is placed on the cranial edge of the vaginal incision in the midline. The clamp is grasped by the surgeon's left hand, and caudad traction is applied while the left index finger

pushes upward (**Fig. 6**). A plane is created that is superficial to the pubocervical fascia through dissection with Metzenbaum scissors at an angle of 60° to 90° to the undersurface of the vaginal incision. The proper plane is identified by noting the characteristic shiny white appearance of the undersurface of the anterior vaginal wall. A small posterior vaginal flap is made for a distance of about 2 cm, just wide enough to accept the sling **Fig. 7** depicts the anatomic relationships between the vaginal wall, pubocervical fascia, and lower urinary tract.

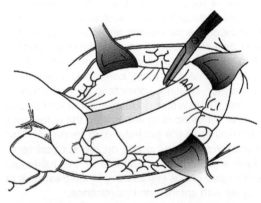

Fig. 3. A plane is created between the fascia and rectus muscle with Mayo scissors, and an index finger places traction on the fascia as the incision is extended superolaterally to the point where the rectus fascia divides to pass around the external oblique muscle. If further length is needed, the incision is extended superiorly. At this point, it is important to avoid the underlying peritoneum. A 2:0 nonabsorbable running horizontal mattress suture is placed across the most lateral portion of the graft. The ends are left long.

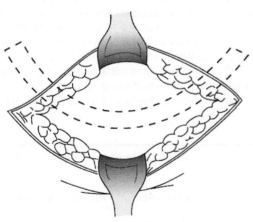

Fig. 2. A 2-cm graft is outlined, keeping the incision parallel to the direction of the fascial fibers.

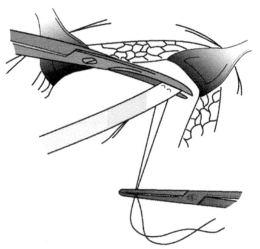

Fig. 4. Each end of the fascial graft is transected approximately 0.5 cm lateral to the mattress suture.

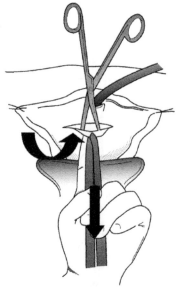

The lateral edges of the wound are grasped with Allis clamps and retracted laterally. The dissection continues just beneath the vaginal epithelium, and Metzenbaum scissors are pointed in the direction of the patient's ipsilateral shoulder (**Fig. 8**) using the index finger (**Fig. 9**) until the periostium of the pubis is palpable. During this part of the dissection, it is important to stay as far lateral as possible to insure that the urethra, bladder, and ureters are

Fig. 6. An Allis clamp is placed on the cranial edge of the vaginal incision in the midline. The clamp is grasped by the surgeon's left hand of the surgeon, and caudad traction is applied while the left index finger pushes upward. A plane is created superficial to the pubocervical fascia by dissecting with Metzenbaum scissors at an angle of 60° to 90° to the undersurface of the vaginal incision. The proper plane is identified by noting the characteristic shiny white appearance of the undersurface of the anterior vaginal wall. A small posterior vaginal flap is made for a distance of about 2 cm, just wide enough to accept the sling.

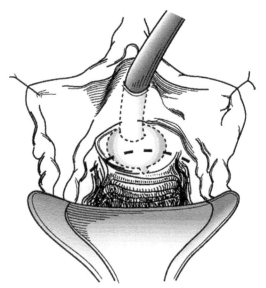

Fig. 5. A 4-cm transverse or slightly curved incision is made in the anterior vaginal wall about 2 cm proximal to the proximal edge of the Foley catheter balloon. This area is the approximate site of the vesical neck. The depth of this incision extends just superficial to the pubocervical fascia.

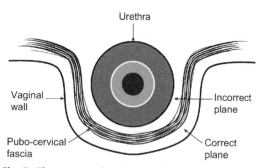

Fig. 7. The proper plane is superficial to the pubocervical fascia. The plane is apparent as the shiny white undersurface of the vaginal wall. If the incision is made deep to the pubocervical fascia, the dissection proceeds just underneath the urethra and bladder, exposing those structures to the possibility of injury. The wrong plane also has a shiny white surface, so great care must be exercised to ensure that the correct plane is identified.

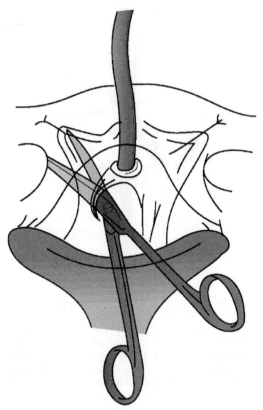

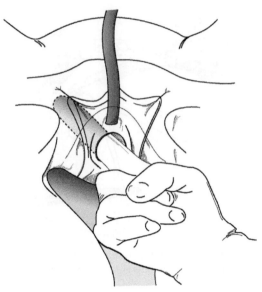

Fig. 9. The endopelvic fascia is perforated with the index finger, and the retropubic space is entered. The bladder neck and proximal urethra bluntly are dissected free of their attachments to the vaginal and pelvic walls.

Fig. 8. The lateral edges of the wound are grasped with Allis clamps and retracted laterally (not pictured). The dissection continues just beneath the vaginal epithelium, and the Metzenbaum scissors are pointed in the direction of the patient's ipsilateral shoulder until the periostium of the pubis is palpable. During this part of the dissection, it is important to stay as far lateral as possible to ensure that the urethra, bladder, and ureters are not injured. This step is accomplished by pointing the concavity of the scissors laterally and by exerting constant lateral pressure with the tips of the scissors against the undersurface of the vaginal epithelium. Once the periostium is reached, the endopelvic fascia is perforated, and the retropubic space is entered.

not injured. This step is accomplished by pointing the concavity of the scissors laterally and by exerting constant lateral pressure with the tips of the scissors against the undersurface of the vaginal epithelium. Once the periostium is reached, the endopelvic fascia is perforated, and the retropubic space is entered. The bladder neck and proximal urethra bluntly are dissected free of their attachments to the vaginal and pelvic walls.

A Kocher clamp is placed on the inferior edge of the rectus fascia in the midline, and the fascia is pulled upward. The left index finger is reinserted into the vaginal wound, retracting the vesical

neck and bladder medially. The tip of the finger palpates the right index finger, which is inserted just beneath the inferior leaf of the rectus fascia and guided along the undersurface of the pubis until it meets the left index finger from the vaginal wound (**Fig. 10**). A long curved clamp (DeBakey) is inserted into the incision and directed to the undersurface of the pubis. The tip of the clamp is pressed against the periostium and directed toward the left index finger, which retracts the vesical neck and bladder medially (**Fig. 11**). At all times, the left index finger is kept between the tip of the clamp and the bladder and urethra, protecting these structures from injury. In this fashion, the clamp is guided into the vaginal wound. When the tip of the clamp is visible in the vaginal wound, the long suture, which is attached to the fascial graft, is grasped and pulled into the abdominal wound (**Fig. 12**). The procedure is repeated on the other side.

Two small stab wounds are made in the rectus fascia just above the pubis (**Fig. 13**), and the sling is brought through them on either side (**Fig. 14**). The fascial sling now is positioned from the abdominal wall on one side, around the undersurface of the vesical neck, and back to the abdominal wall on the other side.

Five milliliters of indigo carmen are given intravenously, and cystoscopy is performed to insure that there is no damage to the urethra, vesical neck, bladder, or ureters. The sling is put on

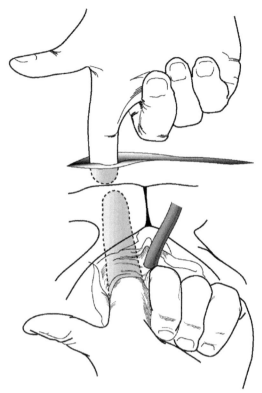

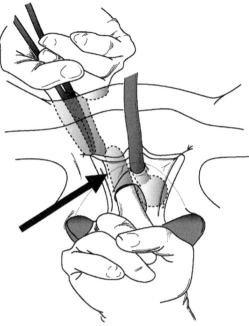

Fig. 10. A Kocher clamp is placed on the inferior edge of the rectus fascia in the midline, and the fascia is pulled upward (not pictured). The left index finger is reinserted into the vaginal wound, retracting the vesical neck and bladder medially. The tip of the finger palpates the right index finger, which is inserted just beneath the inferior leaf of the rectus fascia and guided along the undersurface of the pubis until it meets the left index finger from the vaginal wound.

Fig. 11. A long curved clamp (DeBakey) is inserted into the incision and directed to the undersurface of the pubis. The tip of the clamp is pressed against the periostium and directed toward the left index finger, which retracts the vesical neck and bladder medially. At all times, the left index finger is kept between the tip of the clamp and the bladder and urethra, protecting these structures from injury. In this fashion, the clamp is guided into the vaginal wound.

tension by pulling up on the sutures, and the position of the sling is noted by observing where the urethra coapts. Historically, the sling has been placed intentionally at the bladder neck, and the authors continue to place it there; however, if cystoscopy shows that the sling is distal to the bladder neck, the authors do not attempt to reposition it. The results presented in this article are based on placement of the sling at the vesical neck rather than the midurethra. If cystoscopy shows that the sling inadvertently is placed proximal to the vesical neck, the sling is removed, and a new tunnel is created more distally. The authors generally place a trocar 14-Fr suprapubic tube percutaneously into the bladder, and its position visually is inspected to ensure that it is far away from the trigone. Although this step is not necessary in all patients, the authors find that it facilitates the postoperative voiding trial.

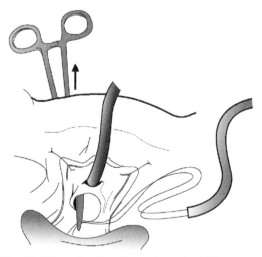

Fig. 12. When the tip of the clamp is visible in the vaginal wound, the long suture, which is attached to the fascial graft, is grasped and pulled into the abdominal wound. The procedure is repeated on the other side. The fascial sling now is positioned from the abdominal wall on one side, around the undersurface of the vesical neck, and back to the abdominal wall on the other side.

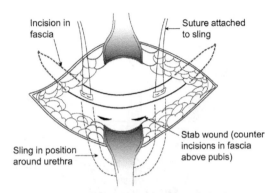

Incision in fascia

Suture attached to sling

Sling in position around urethra

Stab wound (counter incisions in fascia above pubis)

Fig. 13. Two small stab wounds are made in the rectus fascia just above the pubis.

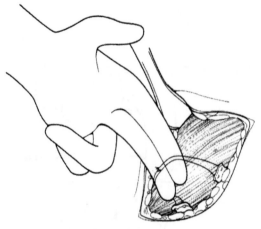

Fig. 15. The wound is closed.

The vaginal incision is closed with running sutures of 2:0 chromic catgut before securing the sling in place. The sutures that are attached to the sling are pulled through the separate stab wounds in the inferior leaf of the rectus fascia on either side (see **Fig. 14**), and the fascial defect is closed with a continuous 2:0 delayed absorbable monofilament suture. The long sutures that are attached to the ends of the fascial graft are tied to one another in the midline, securing the sling in place without any tension (**Fig. 15**).

To insure that excessive tension is not placed on the sling, the authors use several techniques. With the cystoscope in the bladder, the sutures on each end of the fascial strip are grasped and pulled gently upward while downward pressure

is applied to the cystoscope. This approach depresses the vesical neck and puts the sling on stretch. The suture is released, removing excess tension from the sling. The cystoscope is removed, and a well-lubricated Q-tip is placed in the urethra. With the table placed exactly parallel to the floor, the urethral angle is measured. If the angle is negative, downward pressure is placed on the Q-tip at the bladder neck until the angle is 0° or greater. The sutures that are attached to the sling are tied over the rectus fascia with no added tension. It is usually possible to place two fingers comfortably between the sutures and the rectus fascia.

The completed procedure is depicted in **Fig. 16**. A vaginal pack is usually not left unless there has

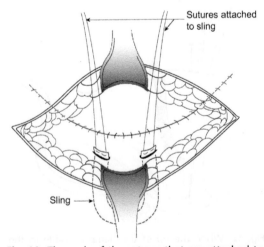

Sutures attached to sling

Sling

Fig. 14. The ends of the sutures that are attached to the sling are pulled through the stab wounds on either side, and the rectus fascia is closed with a 2:0 continuous delayed absorbable monofilament suture. The sutures that are attached to the ends of the fascial graft are tied to one another in the midline, securing the sling in place without tension.

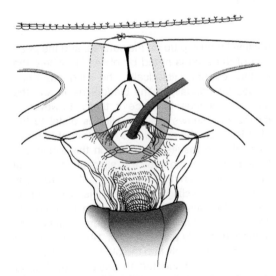

Fig. 16. The completed procedure. The sling is beneath the urethra, and each end is tied to the other over the rectus fascia.

been excessive bleeding. If one is used, it is soaked in sterile lubricating jelly to facilitate its painless removal after surgery.

POSTOPERATIVE MANAGEMENT

If a vaginal pack was used, it is removed the day after surgery. Voiding trials are begun as soon as the patient is comfortable, usually on the first or second postoperative day. If the patient is unable to void by the time of discharge, intermittent self-catheterization is taught.

More than 90% of patients void well enough by 1 week so that intermittent self-catheterization is not necessary, and more than 99% of patients are catheter free by 1 month. Permanent intermittent self-catheterization or urethral obstruction requiring surgery is necessary in less than 1% of patients.

RESULTS

The author's results have been published in four reports over the past 15 years and are summarized.[1–4] Since 1988, all women at our institution who undergo pubovaginal sling have been evaluated by structured history and physical examination, voiding diary, pad test, videourodynamics, and cystoscopy. After surgery, the diaries, pad tests, uroflow, and postvoid residual urine are repeated at each follow-up visit. Use of other outcome instruments, including questionnaires, symptoms scores, and patient-satisfaction indices, has been added over the years. According to the authors, the most accurate tool is the simplified urinary incontinence outcome score (SUIOS).[4] The SUIOS is comprised of three components: a 24-hour voiding diary, 24-hour pad test, and a patient outcome questionnaire, each of which has a range of scores from 0 to 2 points (**Table 1**). Cure (0 points) is defined as

Table 2
Simplified urinary incontinence outcome score (SUIOS)

Outcome	Total Score
Cure	0
Good response	1–2
Fair response	3–4
Poor response	5
Failure	6

a patient's statement that she is cured, a dry pad test, and no incontinence episodes recorded in a voiding diary. Scores of 2 to 5 points are considered improvement, and a score of 6 points is failure (**Table 2**). For the purposes of outcome analysis, the authors divided patients into two groups: simple incontinence and complex incontinence. Complex incontinence was defined as sphincteric incontinence with at least one of the following conditions: urge incontinence, pipe stem urethra (a fixed scarred urethra), urethral or vesicovaginal fistula, urethral diverticulum, grade 3 or 4 cystocele, and neurogenic bladder. In the absence of these conditions, incontinence was considered to be simple.

Overall, the cure–improve rate and fail rate for 325 patients were 93% and 7%, respectively (mean follow-up, 4 years) (**Table 3**). For a subset of 67 patients with uncomplicated incontinence, the cure–improve rate was 100% (**Table 4**). Patients with scores of 5 or 6 points might have been considered to be failures; however, they were considered to have improved because, according to a validated instrument, the patients believed that they had improved despite persistence incontinence. In a separate analysis of 98 women, similar cure–improve and fail rates were found among with stress incontinence and women with mixed incontinence (97% vs 93%,

Table 1
Urinary incontinence survey instruments

Score	0	1	2
24-h diary, Incontinence episodes	0	1–2	≥3
24-h pad test, Weight gain (g)	≤8	9–20	≥21
Patient questionnaire (subjective assessment)	Cure	Improve	Fail

Adapted from Groutz A, Blavias JG, Rosenthal JE. A simplified urinary incontinence score for the evaluation of treatment outcomes. Neurouro Urodyn 2000;19:127–35.

Table 3
SUIOS after pubovaginal sling procedure for simple and complex sphincteric urinary incontinence

Outcome	Total Score	Patients (%)
Cure	0	45
Good response	1–2	27
Fair response	3–4	14
Poor response	5	7
Failure	6	7

Table 4
SUIOS after pubovaginal sling procedure for simple sphincteric urinary incontinence

Outcome	Total Score	Patients (%)
Cure	0	67
Good response	1–2	21
Fair response	3–4	9
Poor response	5	3
Failure	6	0

respectively; $P = 0.33$ using a SUIOS of 4 points as the cutoff between fail and cure or improvement).[3] In that study, patients also were divided into two groups: cured and not cured. Among the patients with mixed incontinence, there was no difference between the cured group and not-cured group with respect to age, surgery, menopausal status, bladder capacity, leak point pressure, pad weight, or type of overactive bladder. Patients who were not cured had more daily preoperative urgency episodes (5.6 vs 4.1 of cured patients) and urge incontinence episodes (5.1 vs 3), and they voided more frequently (12 vs 8 episodes). This finding suggests that the more severe the overactive bladder, the less likely the patient is to respond favorably to surgery.

In the author's combined series, most failures occurred within the first 6 months after surgery, and the most common cause of failure was persistent urge incontinence rather than stress incontinence. De novo urge incontinence occurred in about 3% of their series.

Over the years, significant complications have been uncommon. Only one patient died (an 80-year-old woman as a result of cardiac arrhythmia) in more than 500 patients (<0.2%). Each of the following complications occurred in only 1% of patients: wound infections, incisional hernia, and unexpected long-term urethral obstruction requiring surgery or intermittent catheterization. The authors could not identify any preoperative prognostic factors associated with urinary retention, in no small part because of the fact that it was so uncommon that it would take an enormous number of patients to power a study sufficiently to detect differences. Empirically, there were two causes: grade 3 and grade 4 pelvic organ prolapse, and placing the sling under too much tension. Adjusting tension comes in large part from experience; no long-term urethral obstruction that required surgery or long-term catheterization has occurred in the author's last 300 pubovaginal slings.

DISCUSSION

In a metanalysis of the peer-reviewed English literature, the American Urological Association (AUA) Female Stress Incontinence Clinical Guidelines Panel concluded that with short-term (1-year) and medium-term (4-year) success rates of more than 80%, pubovaginal sling and retropubic suspensions are the most efficacious procedures for treating stress incontinence.[5] Although there was insufficient data to look at subpopulations, it was believed that slings are likely to be more effective in treating intrinsic sphincter deficiency than in retropubic procedures.

In that same study, the investigators decried the paucity of scientifically valid outcome studies and recommended that better outcome instruments be developed and used in prospective trials. Since that report, a number of outcome instruments have been developed (including the SUIOS), and it is hoped that future studies will improve.

Many peer-reviewed studies have corroborated the panel's conclusions (albeit with the same scientific pitfalls) and have reported rates of persistent urge incontinence of 11% to 57% and de-novo urge incontinence rates of 0% to 30%.[1–4,6–17] Urethral obstruction requiring surgery or long-term intermittent catheterization was reported in 1% to 7% of cases. A new AUA guidelines panel is reviewing the literature, and its report is expected within the next few years.

Traditionally, patients have been classified on an anatomic basis (types 0–3) or a functional basis (urethral hypermobility or intrinsic sphincter deficiency), and the type of surgery has been based in part on the classification.[18] The authors no longer use these classification systems, but characterize the incontinence by two parameters: the leak point pressure and the degree of urethral mobility (Q-tip angle). No matter what the type, the authors and other investigators advocate use of the autologous fascial pubovaginal sling.[2,17–19]

SUMMARY

The autologous fascial pubovaginal sling remains the gold standard against which other surgeries for treating sphincteric incontinence should be compared. The authors have demonstrated that this procedure can be performed in a reproducible fashion with minimal morbidity. Using validated objective, semiobjective, and subjective outcome instruments, cure–improve rates of more than 90% have been documented. Urinary retention that occurs after the procedure should be minimal, as the sling is not tied with excessive tension. Persistent and de novo urge incontinence remain vexing problems that the patient should be counseled about before surgery. Although the authors believe that in the future some form of synthetic or allograft sling will be shown to have equal or better efficacy and result in less morbidity, none has yet achieved that status.

REFERENCES

1. Blaivas JG, Jacobs BZ. Pubovaginal fascial sling for the treatment of complicated stress incontinence. J Urol 1991;145:1214.
2. Chaikin DC, Rosenthal J, Blaivas JG. Pubovaginal fascial sling for all types of stress urinary incontinence: long-term analysis. J Urol 1998;160:1312–6.
3. Chou EC, Flisser AJ, Panagopopous G, et al. Effective treatment of mixed urinary incontinence with a pubovaginal sling. J Urol 2003;170:494–7.
4. Groutz A, Blaivas JG, Hyman MJ, et al. Pubovaginal sling surgery for simple stress urinary incontinence: analysis by an outcome score. J Urol 2001;165:1597–600.
5. Leach GE, Dmochowski RR, Appell RA, et al. Female stress urinary incontinence clinical guidelines panel summary report on surgical management of female stress urinary incontinence. J Urol 1997;158:875–80.
6. Barrington JW, Fulford S, Bales G, et al. The modified rectus fascial sling for the treatment of genuine stress incontinence. J Obstet Gynaecol 1998;18:61–2.
7. Carr LK, Walsh PJ, Abraham VE, et al. Favorable outcome of pubovaginal slings for geriatric women with stress incontinence. J Urol 1997;157:125–8.
8. Cross CA, Cespedes RD, McGuire EJ. Our experience with pubovaginal slings in patients with stress urinary incontinence. J Urol 1998;159:1195–8.
9. Fulford SCV, Flynn R, Barrington J, et al. An assessment of the surgical outcome and urodynamic effects of the pubovaginal sling for stress incontinence and the associated urge syndrome. J Urol 1999;162:135–7.
10. Hassouna ME, Ghoniem GM. Long-term outcome and quality of life after modified pubovaginal sling for intrinsic sphincter deficiency. Urology 1999;53:287–91.
11. Kochakarn W, Leenanupunth C, Ratana-Olarn K, et al. Pubovaginal sling for the treatment of female stress urinary incontinence: experience of 100 cases at Ramathibodi Hospital. J Med Assoc Thai 2001;84:1412–5.
12. Kuo HC. Comparison of video urodynamic results after the pubovaginal sling procedure using rectus fascia and polypropylene mesh for stress urinary incontinence. J Urol 2001;165:163–8.
13. McGuire EJ, Lytton B. Pubovaginal sling procedure for stress incontinence. J Urol 1978;119:82–4.
14. McGuire EJ, Bennet CJ, Konnak JA, et al. Experience with pubovoginal slings for urinary incontinence at the University of Michigan. J Urol 1987;138:525.
15. McGuire EJ, Lytton B, Pepe V. Value of urodynamic testing in stress urinary incontinence. J Urol 1980;124:256.
16. Morgan TO, Westney OL, McGuire EJ. Pubovaginal sling: 4-year outcome analysis and quality of life assessment. J Urol 2000;163:1845–8.
17. Zaragoza MR. Expanded indications for the pubovaginal sling: treatment of type 2 or 3 stress incontinence. J Urol 1996;156:1620–2.
18. Blaivas JG, Olsson CA. Stress incontinence: classification and surgical approach. J Urol 1988;139:727–31.
19. Appell RA. Primary slings for everyone with genuine stress incontinence? The argument for…. Int Urogynecol J 1998;9:249–51.

The Treatment of Posterior Compartment Vaginal Defects

R. Duane Cespedes, MD

KEYWORDS

- Posterior compartment prolapse • Rectocele • Enterocele

Posterior compartment prolapse can be thought of as a relaxation or separation of the tissues of the rectovaginal septum and perineal body. Common symptoms include difficulty with defecation and, less commonly, sexual dysfunction. A continued active lifestyle and improved quality of life usually can be restored; however, this result requires a thorough understanding of pelvic anatomy and pathophysiology and experience in performing the appropriate surgical procedures. This article reviews the pathophysiology, diagnosis, and surgical management of rectoceles and relaxed vaginal outlet.

PELVIC FLOOR PHYSIOLOGY

The main support for the pelvic viscera is provided by a group of muscles collectively called the levator ani. An intact pelvic floor allows the pelvic and abdominal viscera to rest on the levator ani, significantly reducing the tension on the supporting fascia and ligaments. These pelvic ligaments are not true ligaments and are condensations of the endopelvic fascia that covers the pelvic structures. The pelvic floor musculature and the pelvic ligaments work together to provide support to the pelvic floor structures. Most of the weight of the pelvic viscera is supported by the levator ani, whereas the pelvic ligaments stabilize these structures in position much like water supports a ship's weight and moorings keep a ship from straying away from the dock.[1] When the levator ani is damaged, excessive force is placed on the ligaments, predisposing the patient to pelvic prolapse.

The posterior vaginal wall in the midvagina is supported centrally and laterally by rectovaginal fascia, which is attached to the fascia of the levator ani musculature. These attachments prevent the rectum from prolapsing into the vagina, causing a rectocele. The distal vagina is attached firmly to the surrounding structures, including the urethra and symphysis pubis anteriorly, levator ani laterally, and perineal musculature posteriorly. Damage to the perineal musculature by childbirth or surgery is a common cause for rectoceles and a relaxed vaginal outlet.

PATHOPHYSIOLOGY

The pathophysiology of posterior vaginal wall relaxation often can be linked to multiparity, advanced age, hormonal insufficiency, obesity, neurogenic dysfunction of the pelvic floor, connective tissue abnormalities, or strenuous physical activity; however, pelvic relaxation can occur in young, inactive, nulliparous patients, and a single cause rarely can be implicated.[2,3] The exact incidence of relaxed vaginal outlet is unknown because not all patients are symptomatic; however, the condition is believed to be common.

A rectocele is a prolapse of the rectum into the vagina through a damaged rectovaginal septum

A version of this article was previously published in the *Atlas of the Urologic Clinics of North America* 12:2.
No funding support was used. The views expressed herein are those of the authors and do not reflect the views of the United States Air Force or Department of Defense.
Department of Urology, Wilford Hall Medical Center, Lackland Air Force Base, TX 78236, USA
E-mail address: dcespedes@satx.rr.com

(Fig. 1). The most likely cause of rectocele formation and perineal relaxation is childbirth, as these conditions are essentially confined to parous women.[4] In some cases, a relaxed outlet may be caused by an inadequate or incompletely healed episiotomy that was performed at the time of childbirth.

The most important fascia within the rectovaginal septum is Denonvilliers fascia, which is fused to the inner layer of the posterior vaginal wall and is believed to be disrupted at the caudal and lateral attachments at the perineal body during childbirth.[5] In some cases, enterocele and rectocele formation occur together, especially if the patient has had a previous hysterectomy. Although a high rectocele may be only distinguished from an enterocele at the time of surgery, a rectocele often forms a pocket just proximal to the anal sphincter. This pocket is where stool can become trapped and can cause the typical symptoms of straining or the need for digital manipulation (splinting) to facilitate bowel movements.[6]

Perineal body relaxation, a separate and distinct entity from a rectocele, usually is manifested by a large vaginal opening and is repaired at the same time as a rectocele. Because the levator ani are attached at the perineal body, strengthening of the perineal body by perineorrhaphy tightens the levator plate, improving the overall degree of pelvic relaxation.

CLINICAL PRESENTATION

The most common symptoms of a rectocele and relaxed outlet are constipation, which is nonspecific, and splinting, which is the need to place fingers on the posterior wall of the vagina to empty the bowels.[7] In general, the larger the relaxation, the more severe the symptoms; however, Caps[8] reported that 8% of symptomatic patients had mild relaxation. Other presenting symptoms may include perineal pain or sexual dysfunction; however, these symptoms are uncommon. Dyspareunia has been reported after a surgical repair in up to 30% of cases. The current incidence is less than 10%, because the older method of repair, which plicated the levator musculature, is now seldom used.[9,10]

INDICATIONS

Rectocele repair is rarely required unless the patient has an anatomic defect and typical constipation symptoms. At my institution, I occasionally repair isolated large rectoceles that cause significant pressure symptoms and repair large rectoceles as a part of an overall vaginal vault prolapse reconstruction. It is difficult to justify postoperative dyspareunia to fix a small, asymptomatic rectocele or perineal body. Some investigators believe that not performing these repairs at the time of an incontinence procedure or

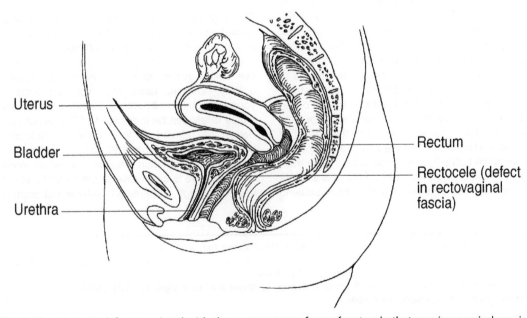

Fig. 1. The anatomic defect associated with the most common form of rectocele that requires surgical repair.

hysterectomy may cause undue pressure on other areas of the pelvic floor, possibly necessitating additional surgery at a later date. This has not been my experience, however.[11]

PHYSICAL EXAMINATION

In many cases, a rectocele easily may be seen when the patient quickly bears down; however, if this position is maintained for only a short period of time, some rectoceles (and an enterocele or vault prolapse) may not be appreciated. Unlike a cystocele evaluation, the rectum cannot be filled, and a digital inspection may be required for further evaluation, especially if the patient is unable to strain sufficiently. A surgical plan should be made before going to the operating room. This evaluation cannot be performed adequately under anesthesia, because the patient is unable to strain and the pelvic muscles are relaxed. The posterior vaginal wall is examined by placing the lower blade of the Graves speculum against the anterior vaginal wall. A bulging of the posterior vaginal wall with straining may be an enterocele or a rectocele (**Fig. 2**). Descent of the vaginal wall at the level of the hymen or below is usually a rectocele,

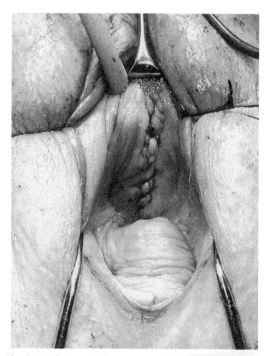

Fig. 2. In this vaginal reconstruction, a large rectocele is located distally and an enterocele is located proximally where the mucosa is smooth. The presence of an enterocele should be anticipated, as additional surgery is required for repair.

whereas prolapse near the apex may be an enterocele. After a hysterectomy, descent of the vaginal apex with straining indicates a lack of vault support. The perineal body, which lies between the vagina and anus, should be evaluated for structural integrity. A lax perineal body usually is manifested by an enlarged introitus or a flattening of the perineum with descent on straining.

IMAGING STUDIES

Imaging studies are not commonly needed for evaluation of symptomatic pelvic prolapse of any type, as the physical examination almost always yields a clear diagnosis and the therapy rarely is altered by additional studies. In some cases in which the patient remains symptomatic after multiple previous procedures have been performed, a dynamic MRI or defecography may be helpful in diagnosing an occult prolapse defect, including a perineal descent syndrome. This syndrome is diagnosed radiographically when the patient strains and the perineum descends past the ischial tuberosities. This condition may be confused with a rectocele and is treated with fixation of the perineal body to the rectocele repair or intact distal pararectal fascia. Endorectal ultrasonography of the anus and rectum may be helpful in diagnosing certain incontinence disorders by imaging the anatomic integrity of the internal and external anal sphincters. Other radiographic studies, such as colonic transit times (for motility issues) and sphincter electromyography (for paradoxic puborectalis contraction), can help with determining why the patient remains symptomatic after a seemingly adequate rectocele repair.

TREATMENT
Preoperative Considerations

The patient is given enemas the night before the procedure to cleanse the rectum, and preoperative intravenous antibiotics are given. Generally, the rectocele and perineal body repair are performed last if other procedures are to be performed, because vaginal exposure is decreased by these repairs.

Intraoperative Details

Some investigators place Betadine-soaked packing into the rectum to assist in identifying the rectum and to avoid injury; however, I use a finger to push the rectum posteriorly to protect it and place the pararectal fascia on tension for suture placement. Placement of a rubber finger in the rectum, as used in a transurethral resection of the prostate, can be helpful for intermittently placing a clean finger into the rectum to evaluate the defects and progress of the repair.

The ultimate size of the vaginal orifice is determined by placing Allis clamps on the inner aspect of the posterior labia and bringing the clamps together. Two or three fingers easily should be admitted. The skin between the Allis clamps is incised, and a triangular skin incision is made on the perineal body with the apex pointing toward the anus. The overlying skin is removed, and the distal vaginal mucosa is infiltrated with saline to facilitate dissection through the typically densely scarred distal tissue. A midline vaginal incision is made that extends at least 1 cm proximal to the beginning of the rectocele (**Fig. 3**). Distal dissection can be difficult; however, once past this area, dissection within the rectovaginal space should proceed easily. If it does not and significant bleeding or repeated perforation of the mucosa occurs, the proper plane has not been found. Once the distal extent of the incision and dissection has been reached, the underlying pararectal fascia is dissected off the posterior vaginal wall until the medial margins of the pubococcygeus muscle are seen (**Fig. 4**). The proximal dissection is easier if the posterior vaginal wall is straightened with a Deaver retractor placed on the anterior vaginal wall with the end of the Deaver retractor placed under the proximal mucosal edge, pulling the vault inward. The fascial dissection should be

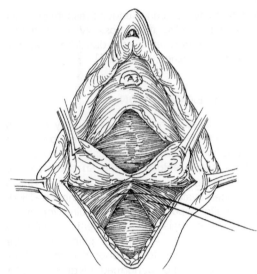

Fig. 4. The rectocele repair is started proximally at least 1 cm above the rectocele defect. The rectum is pushed down, and the fascia is retracted distally using the nondominant hand.

stopped at the lateral fixation of the pararectal fascia, which is seen as the lateral mucosal sulci. If the tissues are weak, it is easy to disrupt this fixation point, and such disruption hampers repair because a posterior lateral defect is created and has to be repaired first.

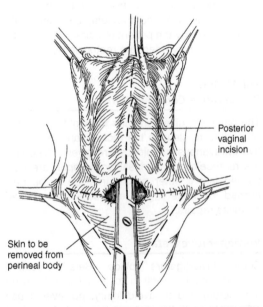

Posterior vaginal incision

Skin to be removed from perineal body

Fig. 3. After sizing of the vaginal opening with Allis clamps, removal of the perineal skin, and infiltration of the mucosa, the posterior vaginal mucosa is opened sharply using Metzenbaum scissors.

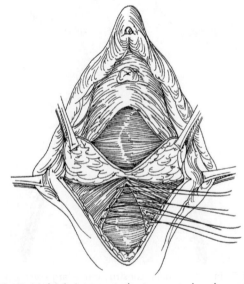

Fig. 5. Multiple interrupted sutures are placed approximately 0.5 cm apart all the way to the perineal body. Sutures should be placed at the edge of the fascia (not laterally) to avoid overtightening of the vagina.

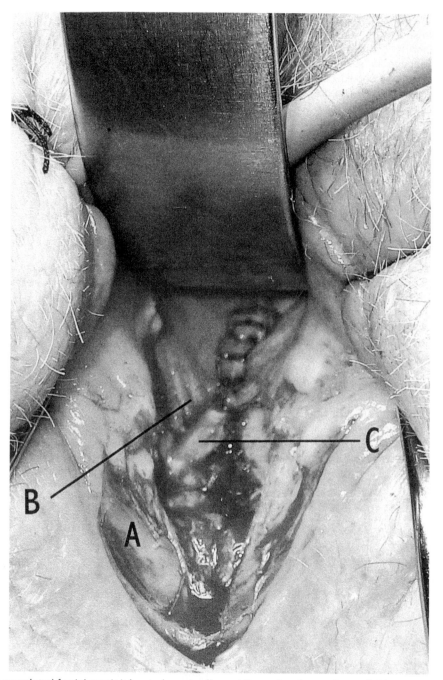

Fig. 6. The completed fascial repair is located proximally, and the perineal musculature (with scar tissue removed) is shown (A). The fascia to be plicated together is seen (C), and the mucosal edge is seen (B).

Starting proximally near the vaginal apex, the pararectal fascia is closed over the rectal wall using absorbable 0 suture (I use 0 Vicryl on a CT-2) in a simple, interrupted fashion that spaces the sutures approximately 0.5 cm apart. The easiest way to place these sutures is to have an assistant retract the anterior wall (for visibility, as described earlier) and to use the left hand (usually just one to two fingers) to push the rectum down and pull the fascia distally, which places it on traction. This approach allows the strong edge of the fascia to be easily seen and helps avoid placing the sutures too far laterally, which can cause overtightening and dyspareunia.

Interrupted sutures are placed sequentially all the way to the perineal body (**Fig. 5**). After the first few sutures are placed, an evaluation easily should allow two fingers to be admitted. If inadequate vaginal caliber is created, dyspareunia or an inability to engage in sexual intercourse may occur. These sutures should be cut out and replaced, as it is much easier to do this step at the time of surgery than to wait and see. The most common reason an inadequate vaginal caliber occurs is that the sutures are placed too far laterally—the sutures should be placed into the edge of the mobile fascia as seen in **Fig. 6** at C. The perineal body is repaired by placing multiple 0 absorbable sutures deeply into the bulbocavernosus and superficial transverse perineal muscles (**Fig. 7**). Two or preferably three fingers should be admitted easily into the vaginal opening. The perineal body is fixated to the distal end of the rectocele repair using a pursestring-type suture placement. This consideration is important, as otherwise the two structures function as separate entities and the perineum can descend, making defecation difficult. This closure minimizes the development of a rectocele between the two repairs. In **Fig. 8**, the distal rectocele repair and proximal edges of the perineal body are marked by asterisks—these tissues need to be fixated together. The vaginal mucosa is closed with an absorbable suture (I use 0 chromic on a CT-2 needle) in a running, locking fashion, and the perineal skin is closed subcuticularly (**Fig. 9**). A vaginal pack is placed to minimize postoperative bleeding in almost all cases.

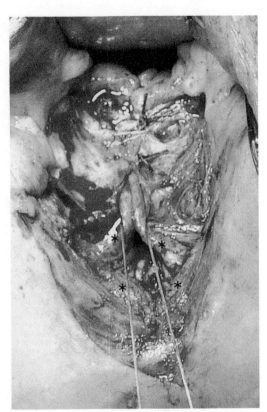

Fig. 8. The distal rectocele repair is shown, as is the perineal musculature that needs to be purse stringed together to ensure adequate fixation of the perineal body to avoid postoperative descent of the perineal body with straining. * The distal rectocele repair and proximal edges of the perineal body.

POSTOPERATIVE CARE

Patients should keep their stools soft, avoid any straining or heavy lifting, and refrain from sexual intercourse for approximately 4 to 6 weeks to allow complete tissue healing.

COMPLICATIONS

Complications are uncommon, and one study reported a 12.5% incidence of transient urinary retention but no rectal injuries, fecal incontinence, or hemorrhage. Dyspareunia can occur after a surgical repair; however, this outcome seems to be uncommon if a sufficient vaginal caliber is maintained. Haase and Skivsted[10] found that approximately 9% of patients experience a deterioration of sexual function after prolapse repairs, but 24% of patients expressed an improvement in sexual satisfaction. The exact incidence of rectal injury is unknown and is probably underreported because most of the injuries easily can be repaired during surgery without long-term

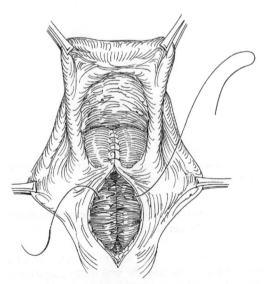

Fig. 7. Repair of the perineal body requires placement of multiple deeply placed sutures into the musculature.

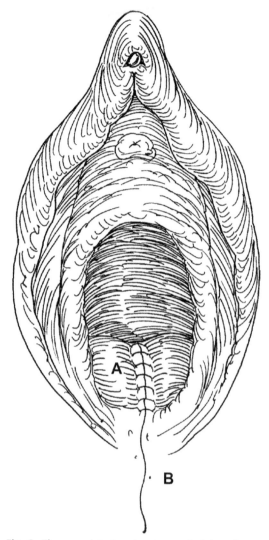

Fig. 9. The completed rectocele repair (A) and perineal body repair at (B).

sequelae. A rectovaginal fistula is a rare complication; however, one study reported a 5% incidence after posterior pelvic floor repairs.[12]

OUTCOME AND PROGNOSIS

Long-term results of rectocele and perineal body repair are unclear, as long-term prospective studies have not been performed. An unpublished retrospective review by Babiarz and Raz[13] reported a 0% failure rate in 95 patients with an unknown length of follow-up. Zimmern et al[14] noted that recurrence is uncommon. At my institution, I have not seen a symptomatic recurrence in more than 225 rectocele repairs. Current thinking is that rectoceles rarely recur after a well-performed rectocele repair.

SUMMARY

A rectocele is a protrusion of the rectum through the attenuated posterior vaginal wall into the lumen of the vagina. Some rectoceles are symptomatic, whereas many rectoceles cause symptoms such as incomplete bowel emptying and vaginal pain and pressure. The treatment of these rectoceles using the diagnostic and therapeutic measures described in this article should provide an excellent outcome in most patients.

REFERENCES

1. DeLancey JOL. Anatomic aspects of vaginal eversion after hysterectomy. Am J Obstet Gynecol 1992;166:1717–28.
2. Norton PA. Pelvic floor disorders: the role of fascia and ligaments. Clin Obstet Gynecol 1993;36:926–38.
3. Wall LL. The muscles of the pelvic floor. Clin Obstet Gynecol 1993;166:910–25.
4. Kuhn RJP, Hollycock VE. Observations on the anatomy of the rectovaginal pouch and septum. Obstet Gynecol 1982;59:445–50.
5. Richardson AC. The anatomic defects in rectocele and enterocele. J Pelvic Surg 1995;1:214–21.
6. Arnold MW, Stewart WR, Aquillar PS. Rectocele repair: four years experience. Dis Colon Rectum 1990;33:684–97.
7. Siproudhis L, Lucas RJ, Raoul JL, et al. Defecatory disorders, anorectal disorders and pelvic floor dysfunction: a polygamy? Int J Colorectal Dis 1992;7:102–7.
8. Caps WR Jr. Rectoplasty and perineoplasty for the symptomatic rectocele: a report of 50 cases. Dis Colon Rectum 1985;18:237.
9. Francis WJA, Jeffcoate TN. Dyspareunia following vaginal operations. Br J Obstet Gynaecol 1961;68:1.
10. Haase P, Skivsted L. Influence of operations for stress incontinence and/or genital decencies on sexual life. Acta Obstet Gynecol Scand 1988;67:659.
11. Nichols DH, Randall CL. Choice of operation for genital prolapse. In: Nichols DH, Randall CL, editors. Vaginal surgery. 4th edition. Baltimore (MD): Lippincott Williams & Wilkins; 1996. p. 130.
12. Pratt JH. Surgical repair of rectocele and perineal lacerations. Clin Obstet Gynecol 1972;15:1160–72.
13. Babiarz JW, Raz S. Pelvic floor relaxation. In: Raz S, editor. Female urology. 2nd edition. Philadelphia: WB Saunders; 1996. p. 456.
14. Zimmern PE, Leach GE, Ganabathi K. The urological aspects of vaginal wall prolapse: Part II. Surgical techniques, complications, and results. AUA Update Series 1993;12:202–7.

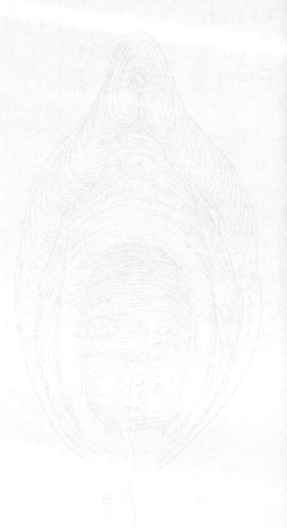

Orthotopic Urinary Diversion in the Female Patient

Emily E. Cole, MD[a], Joseph A. Smith Jr, MD[b],*

KEYWORDS
- Radical cystectomy • Orthotopic reconstruction
- Orthotopic neobladder

The evolution of urinary diversion after radical cystectomy has been impressive over the past century. The ideal form of diversion has yet to be determined, but orthotopic reconstruction offers the most natural voiding pattern, allowing voluntary micturition through the intact native urethra. It has been estimated that more than 50% of patients with invasive bladder cancer are suitable candidates for orthotopic urinary diversion.[1] Before 1990, orthotopic reconstruction was contraindicated in female patients undergoing cystectomy based on two assumptions: (1) Complete removal of the urethra is necessary to provide an adequate surgical margin, and (2) female patients are unable to maintain continence after diversion with an orthotopic neobladder.

Initial concern regarding the possible high urethral recurrence rate has been allayed. Several pathologic reviews have demonstrated that with careful selection of appropriate patients, a portion of the female urethra can be preserved for orthotopic reconstruction.[2–4] These studies determined that tumor involving the bladder neck is the most significant risk factor for urethral tumor involvement; however, approximately 50% of women with tumor at the bladder neck had a urethra that was free of tumor.[2,4] Intraoperative frozen-section analysis of the distal surgical margin (proximal urethra) was found to be an accurate and reliable means for evaluation of the proximal urethra and is the recommended selection criteria for performing an orthotopic diversion in female patients.[5] Because the final decision about the use of orthotopic diversion to the urethra can be influenced by the results of intraoperative frozen sections, patients should be advised of alternative diversion methods before surgery.

Initial concerns about the integrity of the female continence mechanism in cases of urethra-sparing cystectomy also have been allayed. A more comprehensive understanding of the female urethra and continence mechanism has been gained through anatomic and histologic studies of the female pelvis. A transition from smooth muscle to striated muscle in the midurethra to the distal third of the urethra has been described.[6,7] Performing minimal dissection anteriorly and avoiding injury of the pudendal innervation to the rhabdosphincter is crucial in maintaining the midurethral continence mechanism in female patients with neobladders. Maintenance of the urethral support structures may contribute to preserving continence. Preservation of the endopelvic fascia and the pubourethral ligament anterior to the bladder neck and rhabdosphincter is important in maintaining the appropriate anatomic relationships as the urethra courses across the pelvic floor. This support system is augmented by the infrapelvic fascia (levator ani and pubococcygeus muscles) and by the connective supporting tissues of the anterior vaginal wall surrounding the urethra.

A version of this article was previously published in the *Atlas of the Urologic Clinics of North America* 12:2.
[a] Department of Urology, Uniformed Services, University of the Health Sciences, Naval Medical Center, San Diego 34800, Bob Wilson Drive, San Diego, CA 92134, USA
[b] Department of Urologic Surgery, Vanderbilt University Medical Center, A-1302 Medical Center North, Nashville, TN 37232, USA
* Corresponding author.
E-mail address: joseph.smith@vanderbilt.edu

Urol Clin N Am 38 (2011) 25–29
doi:10.1016/j.ucl.2010.12.004

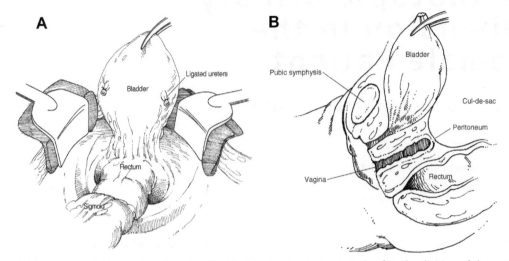

Fig. 1. (*A*) Exposure of the pouch of Douglas. The bladder is retracted anteriorly after the division of the ureters and lateral pedicles exposing the cul-de-sac. (*B*) Lateral view of the pouch of Douglas. The location of the vaginal apex should be noted.

Dissection of the cystectomy specimen off of the anterior vaginal wall may assist in maximizing preservation of support structures and innervation to the anterior urethra, factors that may be important in maintaining passive and voluntary urinary control.[8,9]

Known complications of orthotopic neobladder substitution in females are incomplete voiding and neobladder–vaginal fistula. Urinary retention largely has been attributed to posterior displacement of the pouch with acute urethrointestinal angulation.[10–12] Reported neobladder–vaginal fistulae were found in areas where the vaginal closure suture line overlapped suture lines of the neobladder. The incidence of both of these complications can be decreased by the use of an anterior vaginal-wall–sparing approach to cystectomy.

Knowledge that the urethra and continence mechanism can be preserved safely in female patients undergoing cystectomy has enabled orthotopic lower urinary reconstruction to become a viable and preferred method of diversion at many centers. The authors advocate an anterior vaginal-wall–sparing technique for cystectomy with orthotopic diversion. They believe that this approach achieves adequate oncologic results while preserving necessary support structures and possibly decreasing the incidence of certain complications.

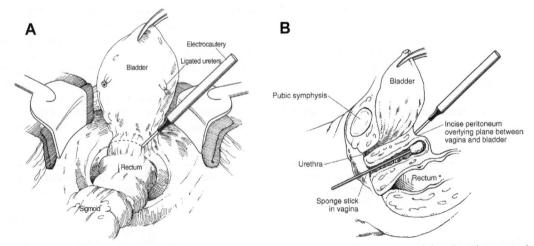

Fig. 2. (*A*) A sponge stick is placed in the vagina and elevated cephalad. The location of the plane between the bladder and the vagina is identified and the overlying peritoneum is incised with electrocautery. (*B*) Incising peritoneum overlying plane between bladder and vagina – lateral view.

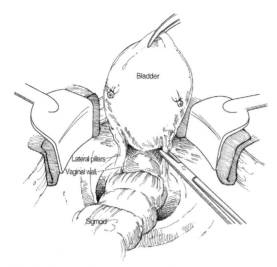

Fig. 3. Central plane between the posterior bladder and vagina has been developed. Remaining lateral attachments are taken down with a vessel-sealing device.

PREOPERATIVE PREPARATION

Female patients who are considered to be candidates for orthotopic neobladder substitution after cystectomy should meet criteria for an anterior vaginal-wall–sparing approach. Patients should undergo preoperative bimanual pelvic examination to allay any suspicion for direct invasion into the vaginal wall. CT scan of the abdomen and pelvis may be helpful to rule out evidence of direct invasion into the reproductive organs. Metastatic evaluation should be performed in all patients according to standards.

TECHNIQUE

The superior, posterior, and lateral pedicles of the bladder are isolated and ligated to the level of the anterior vaginal wall using a right angle and ties or locking surgical clips (**Fig. 1**). A sponge stick is placed in the vaginal vault and elevated cephalad to assist in identification of the apex and anterior wall of the vagina. The bladder is elevated to reveal the peritoneal cul-de-sac, where the impression of the sponge stick can be palpated. The approximate location of the plane between the anterior vaginal wall and the posterior bladder is identified, and the overlying peritoneum is incised with electrocautery (**Fig. 2**). If present, the uterus may be preserved, in which case the plane to be developed is located just caudad to the cervix. If the patient wants to undergo a hysterectomy, the cervix is excised completely. The open ends of the vaginal apex are approximated with absorbable Vicryl suture. The authors recommend that a flap of omentum be secured to cover the oversewn vaginal apex, eliminating the possibility of overlapping suture lines. With continued cephalad elevation of the vaginal wall, the central plane between bladder and vagina is developed with a combination of sharp and blunt dissection. Lateral attachments can be taken down with the assistance of a vessel-sealing ligasure device (**Fig. 3**). Careful dissection in this plane is paramount to avoid inadvertent entry into the specimen or injury to the vaginal wall. The bladder specimen is elevated out of the pelvis as this carefully developed posterior plane is continued to the level of the bladder neck (**Fig. 4**). Palpation of the Foley catheter balloon in the bladder helps to identify

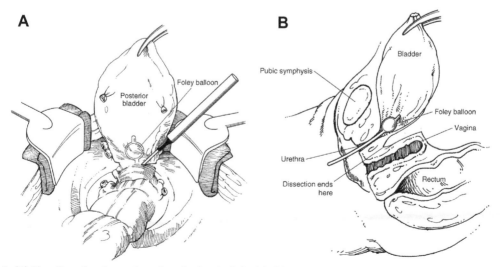

Fig. 4. (A) The dissection is continued to the level of the bladder neck. (B) Lateral view of the continued dissection. The distal extent of dissection should be noted.

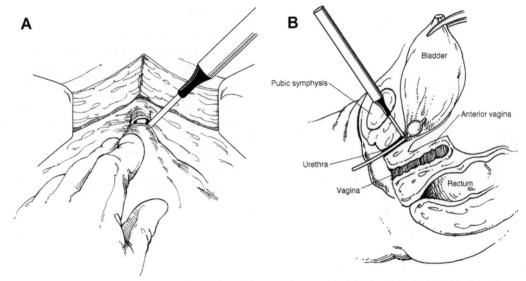

Fig. 5. (*A*) The bladder is lowered into the field, and the anterior urethra is incised just distal to the bladder neck. (*B*) Lateral view of the transection of the urethra.

this stopping point. Any additional distal dissection is discouraged because of the potential disruption of the musculofascial support or innervation of the rhabdosphincteric complex. Attention then is directed to the anterior dissection. Minimal dissection should be performed anteriorly to prevent injury to the distal sphincteric mechanism. The bladder neck can be identified by palpation of the Foley catheter balloon, and an incision is made just distal to this area, exposing the Foley catheter (**Fig. 5**). The urethra is incised completely, and any remaining fibromuscular tissue that is attached to the urethra or perineal body is divided, freeing the specimen for removal. The endopelvic fascia anterior to the rhabdosphincter is not disturbed (**Fig. 6**). Bleeding from the dorsal vein is usually minimal and can be controlled with suture ligatures placed anterior to the urethra. Absorbable sutures are used to control collateral vaginal wall bleeding that cannot be stopped adequately with

electrocautery. The posterior bed of resection is inspected carefully to ensure that no defects in the anterior vaginal wall have been created. Incidental incisions are closed primarily in multiple layers with absorbable Vicryl suture. If possible, a flap of omentum should be secured over the repair to discourage fistula formation. The neobladder is created in accordance with surgeon preference, and 45 to 60 cm of small intestine usually is employed. The authors' preferred configuration is a W-shaped pouch that provides a good-capacity spherical reservoir. Five to six 2-0 Vicryl sutures that are placed circumferentially

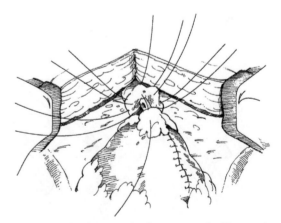

Fig. 7. Neobladder–urethral anastomosis. Five to six 2-0 vicryl sutures that are placed circumferentially around the urethral stump are used to anchor the most dependent segment of the constructed neobladder to the urethra.

Fig. 6. Urethral stump. The intact endopelvic fascia and pubourethral ligaments should be noted.

around the urethral stump are used to anchor the most dependent segment of the constructed neobladder to the urethra (**Fig. 7**).

POSTOPERATIVE CARE AND FOLLOW-UP

Postoperative care should be individualized; however, a treatment pathway serves as a general guideline for perioperative management at the authors' institution. Ureteral stents are removed sequentially before discharge between postoperative days 5 and 7, and the urethral catheter is left in place for 3 weeks; a separate percutaneous catheter is not placed. Postoperative irrigations are begun on postoperative day 2, and patients are taught how to perform these irrigations before being discharged. At 3 weeks after surgery, the urethral catheter is removed. A cystogram is not routinely obtained.

SUMMARY

The previously described technique has produced good results at the authors' institution. The modifications from standard female cystectomy may serve to improve functional outcomes and quality of life. Leaving the anterior vaginal wall intact preserves some elements of pelvic support and helps to maintain the appropriate anatomic relationships as the urethra courses across the pelvic floor. Most of the authors' patients have reported adequate continence with minimal pad usage, and few patients have experienced problems with urinary retention. Preservation of the vagina provides obvious advantages for women who remain sexually active.

Early in the authors' series, a single neobladder–vaginal fistula occurred in a patient whose anterior vaginal wall was incised and repaired during dissection. No tissue could be secured between the repair and the neobladder. This situation emphasizes the importance of the interposition of an omental pedical or a peritoneal flap over any repaired vaginal injuries to avoid overlapping suture lines and to decrease the potential for fistula formation.

The authors have been able to perform vaginal-wall–sparing cystectomy without compromising surgical margins in all candidates, including patients with pT3b disease. There is potential for local recurrence, however, warranting continued postoperative follow-up with imaging and physical examination.

Because of their positive results, the authors perform this vaginal-wall–sparing technique in all female patients undergoing cystectomy with orthotopic neobladder substitution. They continue to explore modifications of traditional techniques to improve functional outcomes without sacrificing oncologic control.

REFERENCES

1. Studer UE, Zingg EJ. Ileal orthotopic bladder substitutes. Urol Clin North Am 1997;24:781–93.
2. Stein JP, Cote RJ, Freeman JA, et al. Indications for lower urinary reconstruction in women after cystectomy for bladder cancer: a pathological review of female cystectomy specimens. J Urol 1995;154:1329–33.
3. Stenzl A, Draxl H, Posch B, et al. The risk of urethral tumors in female bladder cancer: can the urethra be used for orthotopic reconstruction of the lower urinary tract? J Urol 1995;153:950–5.
4. Stein JP, Esrig D, Freeman JA, et al. Prospective pathological analysis of female cystectomy specimens: risk factors for orthotopic diversion in women. Urology 1998;51:951–5.
5. Stein JP, Ginsberg DA, Skinner DG. Indications and technique of the orthotopic neobladder in women. Urol Clin North Am 2002;29:725–35.
6. Colleselli K, Stenzl A, Eder R, et al. The female urethral sphincter: a morphological and topographical study. J Urol 1998;160:49–54.
7. Borirakchanyavat S, Aboseif SR, Carroll PR, et al. Continence mechanism of the isolated female urethra: an anatomical study of the intrapelvic somatic nerves. J Urol 1997;158:822–6.
8. Blute ML, Gburek BM. Continent orthotopic urinary diversion in female patients: early Mayo Clinic experience. Mayo Clin Proc 1998;73:501–7.
9. Chang SS, Cole EE, Cookson MS, et al. Preservation of the anterior vaginal wall during female radical cystectomy with orthotopic urinary diversion: technique and results. J Urol 2002;168:1442–5.
10. Hautmann RE, Paiss T, de Petriconi R. The ileal neobladder in women: 9 years of experience with 18 patients. J Urol 1996;155:76–81.
11. Shimogaki H, Okada H, Fujisawa M, et al. Long-term experience with orthotopic reconstruction of the lower urinary tract in women. J Urol 1999;161:573–7.
12. Ali-El-Dein B, El-Sobky E, Hohenfellner M, et al. Orthotopic bladder substitution in women: functional evaluation. J Urol 1999;161:1875–80.

Urethrolysis

Howard B. Goldman, MD

KEYWORDS

- Iatrogenic urethral obstruction
- Urethrolysis • Resuspension

Urethral obstruction after surgery to treat stress urinary incontinence (SUI) is reported to occur in 5% to 20% of patients. Studies report that the incidence of surgery for treating SUI has increased dramatically over the past decade.[1] If only patients requiring an inpatient admission are taken into account, the rate increases by 45%. As most of these procedures are done in the outpatient setting, this figure vastly underestimates the true increase. With this increase in the number of procedures performed, there likely also has been an increase in the number of patients with iatrogenic urethral obstruction. Surgeons who perform these procedures should be adept at recognizing the signs of iatrogenic obstruction and be comfortable with performing a procedure to unobstruct the patient or with referring the patient to someone with more experience in this area. In most cases, timely recognition and treatment lead to significant symptom relief.

MECHANISMS OF OBSTRUCTION

Although an aggressive cystocele repair or other type of pelvic surgery occasionally can lead to iatrogenic urethral obstruction, most cases result from procedures for stress urinary incontinence. Retropubic bladder neck suspensions (BNS), transvaginal suspensions, and traditional bladder neck or midurethral slings can obstruct the urethra.

With a retropubic BNS, the sutures elevating the bladder neck may be too tight or too close to the urethra, or exuberant scarification may have occurred between the pubis and urethra. This situation can lead to kinking and compression of the urethra, resulting in obstruction. A similar mechanism may occur with a transvaginal BNS.

With a sling, there is typically less scarring anterior to the urethra. Not much dissection usually is done anterior to the urethra or between the urethra and the pubis. Most scarring occurs in a more lateral area where the sling perforates the endopelvic fascia. In most obstructing slings, the cause of the obstruction likely is unrelated to anterior or lateral scarification and more likely is related to ventral compression of the urethra by the sling. This concept is supported by the fact that simple division of the sling beneath the urethra, which sometimes is accompanied by stripping of the edges of the sling from the ventral surface of the urethra, usually resolves the problem.[2–5] Although these problems can be related to tying a sling too tight, other unclear patient characteristics or exuberant scarring may lead to obstruction, even in cases in which the sling appeared to be loosely tied. Even the most experienced surgeon runs into this problem on occasion.

PATIENT EVALUATION

Patients with iatrogenic urethral obstruction may present with obstructive or irritative symptoms. Patients who are in retention or complain of markedly diminished force of urinary stream after surgery are easy to identify. Some patients may have more subtle symptoms. Bending forward to void or having to change positions to effectively void usually indicates an element of obstruction. Recurrent urinary tract infections that are associated with an elevated postvoid residual may suggest obstruction. Irritative symptoms, such as new-onset or worsened urgency, urge incontinence, or urinary frequency, may result from the bladder's response to obstruction. Although conservative measures (ie, anticholinergic medication

A version of this article was previously published in the *Atlas of the Urologic Clinics of North America* 12:2.
Center for Female Pelvic Medicine and Reconstructive Surgery, Glickman Urologic and Kidney Institute, The Cleveland Clinic Lerner College of Medicine, Case Western Reserve University, 9500 Euclid Avenue/Q10, Cleveland, OH 44195, USA
E-mail address: goldmah@ccf.org

urologic.theclinics.com

or pelvic floor exercises) may help relieve these symptoms, the possibility of obstruction must be entertained.

The most crucial part of the history is the temporal relationship between surgery and the onset of these symptoms. When a patient complains of new-onset obstructive or irritative symptoms after anti-incontinence surgery, iatrogenic obstruction should be suspected.

On physical examination, hypersuspension of the urethra may be identified. The anterior vaginal wall in the area of the bladder neck may be difficult to visualize and may be fixed to the undersurface of the pubis. During a Q-tip test, the Q-tip may have to be guided over a bump to pass it into the bladder, and a resulting negative (downward) deflection of the tip frequently is noted. On cystoscopy, a ridge at the point of obstruction may be visualized. The previous findings less commonly are noted in obstruction caused by midurethral synthetic slings. Although these signs may help solidify the diagnosis of obstruction, their absence does not rule it out.

Urodynamics can be performed and often demonstrates outflow obstruction. Because many women void with low detrusor pressures, the obstructed state may not cause a significantly elevated detrusor pressure and may not give a classic picture of obstruction. Previous studies have found that outcomes after urethrolysis do not depend on urodynamic findings.[6]

Ultimately, patients with a clear temporal relationship between onset of symptoms and anti-incontinence surgery should be considered for urethrolysis. A corroborating physical examination or urodynamic evidence can further solidify the decision.

CHOICE OF PROCEDURES

There are a number of ways to free up the obstructed urethra. A urethrolysis can be performed transvaginally or from an open retropubic approach. With a transvaginal approach, one can start ventral to the urethra and dissect laterally and anteriorly through the endopelvic fascia and between the anterior surface of the urethra and the pubis. Alternatively, one can incise above the urethra and directly separate it from its anterior attachments. A combination of these transvaginal techniques may be required to fully free the urethra. The less invasive technique of sling incision has been described. Wrapping a Martius flap around the urethra at the time of urethrolysis is another option, and although most surgeons reserve this approach for patients with recurrent

obstruction, some surgeons have advocated its use in primary procedures.[7]

The approach used depends on the type of incontinence surgery that led to the obstruction, whether urethrolysis has been attempted in the past, and whether the surgeon is comfortable with the various approaches.

For patients who previously underwent a sling procedure, regardless of whether the sling was placed at the bladder neck or midurethral, a sling incision may be attempted first. If that approach fails to provide adequate release during surgery or if the patient has recurrent problems, a traditional transvaginal urethrolysis should be performed. Cutting the sling sutures from above and not addressing the ventral obstruction caused by the sling itself are unlikely to be helpful. Within a few weeks, the ends of the sling scar into the retropubic space and cutting the sutures above does not release the sling. After a transvaginal BNS, a traditional transvaginal approach is usually the procedure of choice. Some investigators have advocated a suprameatal, transvaginal approach, suggesting that because the endopelvic fascia remains intact, there is less hypermobility and incontinence after urethrolysis.[8]

For patients with recurrent symptoms after a transvaginal approach, a repeat transvaginal approach with a Martius fat graft is reasonable. Extension to include a suprameatal approach may be necessary. After a failed transvaginal approach, a retropubic approach also may be a good choice and allow better access to retropubic sutures and scar tissue.

If the inciting surgery was a retropubic BNS, a transvaginal or retropubic approach may be attempted.[9] It may be hard to cut all of the sutures or adhesions transvaginally. Although a retropubic approach entails an abdominal incision, it allows full and unimpeded access to all retropubic sutures and scar tissue.

URETHROLYSIS TECHNIQUE
Sling Incision

The patient is placed in a steep Trendelenburg position and positioned in a standard fashion for vaginal surgery. Because of hypersuspension, the bladder-neck area can be difficult to visualize in patients who had a traditional bladder neck sling. A 19-Fr cystoscope sheath or Lowsley retractor is placed within the urethra and gently torqued upward, placing tension on the sling and allowing for easy identification of the constricting band (sling) (**Fig. 1**). A vertical incision is made through the vaginal wall over the sling. With careful blunt and sharp dissection, the sling is identified,

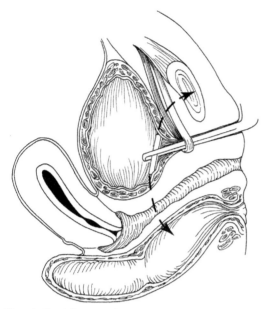

Fig. 1. Straight Lowsley retractor with wings deployed positioned at the bladder neck. The retractor can be moved up and down, side to side, and pivoted against the pubic bone to move the urethra and put tension on the sling.

and the cystoscopy sheath is changed for a Foley catheter.

For patients who had a midurethral synthetic sling, an incision is made about 2.5 cm proximal to the urethral meatus, after which the rough edges of the mesh are usually palpable, and the sling is identified (**Fig. 2**).

With either type of sling, a right-angle clamp carefully is insinuated into the plane between the sling and urethra. Once completely behind the sling, the tips of the right-angle clamp are gently spread wide, leaving a portion of the sling elevated and separate from the urethra. The sling is cut with scissors or a scalpel (**Figs. 3** and **4**). The cut edges usually retract because the tension has been released. I typically make no additional effort to free the sling lateral to the urethra; however, other investigators suggest dissecting to the level of the endopelvic fascia and excising the sling ends.[3] The vaginal wall is closed, and the patient is discharged the same day without a catheter.

Retropubic Urethrolysis

The patient is placed supine on the operating table with the legs slightly spread apart (to allow for manual vaginal access). A lower-midline or Pfannenstiel incision is made. The retropubic space is entered. All visible and palpable suspension sutures are cut, and all scar tissue between the

urethra and pubis is incised sharply (**Fig. 5**). Careful attention is paid to the location of the Foley catheter and balloon to avoid inadvertent bladder or urethral injury. In some cases, there is so much scarring that the bladder can be entered accidentally on entry into the space of Retzius. If this situation occurs, it is helpful to leave the bladder open until the dissection is complete to give a constant sense of where the bladder is in relation to the scar tissue. Placing a finger inside the bladder can be helpful in these cases. Although it is not usually necessary to enter the bladder, one may take advantage of this situation by obtaining an additional sense of geography. It is also useful to palpate the anterior vaginal wall vaginally while incising the scar tissue to maintain a sense of the area that is being dissecting. At the end of the dissection, the urethra, bladder neck, and anterior vaginal wall should be mobilized completely and freed from the pubic bone. One should be able to pass fingers under the pubis and almost see them pushing the vaginal skin out in the distal vagina. At this point, many investigators recommend closing the paravaginal defect created by the dissection. An omental flap can be brought down and fixed so that recurrent scarring between the urethra and pubis is avoided.

Transvaginal Technique

The patient is placed in a lithotomy position with the legs supported by Allen or candy cane stirrups. The lower abdomen and vagina are prepped and draped, and the bed is positioned in steep Trendelenburg position. A Foley catheter is placed. A midline or inverted "U" shaped incision in the anterior vaginal wall is made proximal to the bladder neck and out to the midurethra. Dissection proceeds laterally along the periurethral fascia to the level of the endopelvic fascia, which then is perforated. Any scar tissue or sutures are incised sharply (**Fig. 6**). The anterior surface of the urethra is separated completely from the overlying pubic bone. This step is accomplished with sharp and blunt dissection. A right-angle clamp may be used to bring a suspension suture into view so it can be cut safely. The operative record of the original procedure should be reviewed. If nonabsorbable sutures were used, it is crucial to make sure that all of these sutures are cut. Some separation of the urethra from the pubis is done blindly with Metzenbaum scissors. The surgeon should stay close to the undersurface of the pubis, manually palpate the area of dissection, and be aware of the location of the urethral catheter to avoid inadvertent entry into the urethra or anterior bladder wall near the bladder neck. If either area is entered,

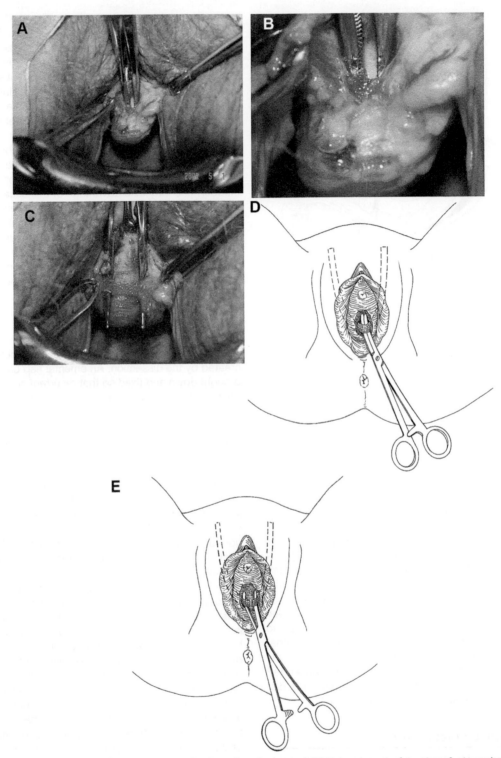

Fig. 2. (*A*) Anterior vaginal wall incision with edge of mesh exposed. (*B*) Enlargement of *A*—tips of scissors behind mesh. (*C*) Synthetic mesh sling fully exposed and ready to be cut. (*D*) Mesh undermined and exposed. (*E*) Mesh transected.

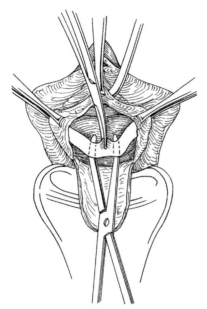

Fig. 3. After an inverted U-shaped or midline incision is made, the sling is isolated in the midline and incised. A right-angle clamp may be placed between the sling and the peri-urethral fascia to avoid injury to the urethra.

careful completion of the procedure should be attempted, avoiding further bladder or urethral wall damage and leaving an indwelling Foley catheter for 2 to 3 weeks. There is little chance of fistula formation, because the area of perforation is well away from the vaginal incision. Heavy bleeding in this area may occur. In this situation, one should expeditiously complete the procedure, close the vaginal wall, and leave a vaginal pack in place. The anterior urethra and bladder neck should be inspected with a cystoscope at the end of the procedure. If an injury is noted, the catheter is

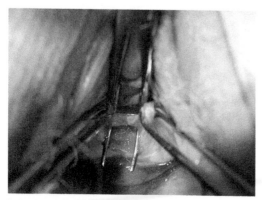

Fig. 4. Fascial sling undermined and ready to be incised.

left in place. If all is intact, the catheter can be removed at the end of the procedure.

If it is difficult to incise all of the scar tissue or suture with this technique a suprameatal incision can be made, and the procedure can be completed in that manner. If dense adhesions are encountered or if this surgery is a repeat procedure, a Martius flap may be wrapped around the urethra to prevent rescarification between the urethra and pubis. Some investigators advocate use of this approach in primary procedures.

Suprameatal Technique

The suprameatal technique can be done as part of the traditional transvaginal urethrolysis or by itself. A semilunar incision is made from the 3 o'clock to 9 o'clock position 1 cm above the urethral meatus (**Fig. 7**). Allis clamps are placed to retract both edges of the incision. With tension on the upper edge, the perineal membrane is perforated, and all attachments, scars, and sutures between the urethra and pubic bone are incised sharply with Metzenbaum scissors. The surgeon's index finger is placed through this area into the retropubic space. Using a sweeping motion laterally and downward, other obstructing bands can be identified and divided sharply or bluntly. If obstruction was secondary to a sling, dissection should be carried laterally until the wings of the sling are identified. They and any suspending sutures then are divided sharply. Once mobilization of the urethra has been accomplished, the original incision is closed with absorbable sutures. Cystourethroscopy should be performed to identify inadvertant urethral or bladder damage.

RESUSPENSION

Performance of resuspension at the time of urethrolysis is controversial. Outcome studies have demonstrated a similar risk for recurrent SUI whether or not resuspension is performed at the time of urethrolysis.[10] If symptoms do not resolve, it is difficult to ascertain whether this situation resulted from an inadequate urethrolysis or obstruction from the resuspension. For these two reasons, I do not perform a routine resuspension at the time of urethrolysis. Only in select patients with SUI before urethrolysis is a concomitant sling or suspension considered.

OUTCOMES

Most large studies on urethrolysis report a success rate of approximately 70% to 80%.[2,3,6-13] Significant symptom relief can be achieved in most patients undergoing repeat urethrolysis after

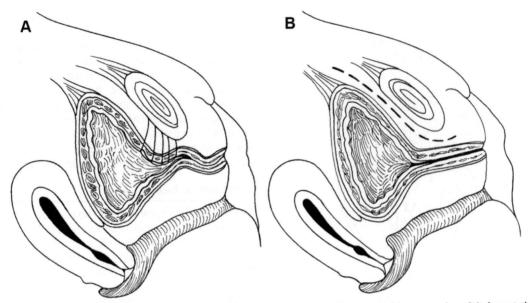

Fig. 5. (*A*) Retropubic urethrolysis. Lateral view of pelvis after obstructive retropubic suspension. Stitches at the level of the bladder neck evaluate and distort the urethrovesical junction, leading to obstruction. (*B*) Lateral view of pelvis after retropubic urethrolysis. Stitches have been removed, and scar tissue has been excised. The dotted line indicates freedom of mobility between the urethra and symphysis pubis. This area is also the location for the placement of an omental interposition graft.

a failed initial attempt.[11] Although most patients have complete or significant relief of obstructive symptoms, it is not unusual that many patients may be left with mild irritative symptoms, albeit they are much improved from their state before

urethrolysis. Heavy bleeding or entry into the bladder neck or urethra may occur during urethrolysis. Closure of any easily accessible lacerations and 2 to 3 weeks of catheter drainage for those that are not accessible usually enable complete

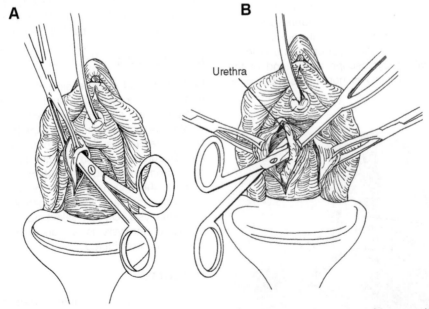

Fig. 6. (*A*) Inverted U-shaped incision in anterior vaginal wall and entrance into retropubic space. (*B*) Urethra is dissected sharply off of the undersurface of the pubic bone. Urethropelvic ligament, periurethral fascia, and vaginal wall are retracted medially to expose urethra in retropubic space.

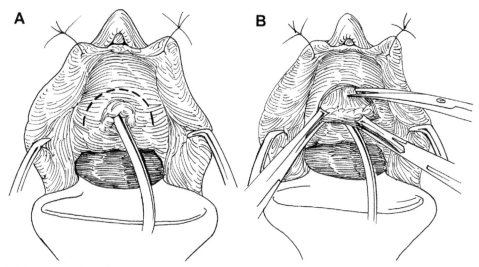

Fig. 7. (*A*) Suprameatal urethrolysis. An inverted U-shaped incision is made superior to the urethral meatus. (*B*) Dissection is performed sharply to the level of the bladder neck. Adhesions between the urethra and symphysis pubis are released.

healing. In the case of bleeding, rapidly finishing the procedure and packing the vagina should allow the bleeding to tamponade and stop.

Recurrent SUI occurs in up to 20% of patients. When it does occur, injection of a bulking agent may prove to be successful in treating incontinence. If that approach fails, a resuspension or sling can be performed after the patient is reevaluated fully.

REFERENCES

1. Waetjen LE, Subak LL, Shen H, et al. Stress urinary incontinence surgery in the United States. Obstet Gynecol 2003;101:67–676.
2. Goldman HB. Simple sling incision for the treatment of iatrogenic urethral obstruction. Urology 2003;62: 714–8.
3. Nitti VW, Carlson KV, Blaivas JG, et al. Early results of pubovaginal sling lysis by midline sling incision. Urology 2002;59:47–51.
4. Klutke C, Siegel S, Carlin B. Urinary retention after tension-free vaginal tape procedure: incidence and treatment. Urology 2001;58:697–701.
5. Kusuda L. Simple release of pubovaginal sling. Urology 2001;57:358–9.
6. Nitti VW, Raz S. Obstruction following anti-incontinence procedures: diagnosis and treatment with transvaginal urethrolysis. J Urol 1994;152: 93–8.
7. Carey JM, Chon JK, Leach GE. Urethrolysis with martius labial fat pad graft for iatrogenic bladder outlet obstruction. Urology 2003;61:21–5.
8. Petrou SP, Brown JA, Blaivas JG. Suprameatal transvaginal urethrolysis. J Urol 1999;161:1268–71.
9. Gomelsky A, Nitti VW, Dmochowski RR. Management of obstructive voiding dysfunction after incontinence surgery: lessons learned. Urology 2003;62: 391–9.
10. Goldman HB, Rackley R, Appell RA. The efficacy of urethrolysis without resuspension for iatrogenic urethral obstruction. J Urol 1999;161:196–9.
11. Scarpero HM, Dmochowski RR, Nitti VW. Repeat urethrolysis after failed urethrolysis for iatrogenic obstruction. J Urol 2003;169:1013–6.
12. Petrou SP, Young PR. Rate of recurrent stress urinary incontinence after retropubic urethrolysis. J Urol 2002;167:613–5.
13. Amundsen CL, Guralnick ML, Webster GD. Variations in strategy for the treatment of urethral obstruction after a pubovaginal sling procedure. J Urol 2000;164:434–7.

The Tension-Free Vaginal Tape Procedure

Steven D. Kleeman, MD[a,b,*], Mickey M. Karram, MD[c,d]

KEYWORDS

- Suburethral slings • Transvaginal approach
- Suprapubic approach

The first sling operation was reported by Von Giordano in 1907. Von Giordano used a gracilis muscle flap in a patient with epispadias.[1] In 1970, the Goebell-Frankenheim-Stoekel procedure was described during which the perimedalis muscle and rectus fascia was plicated beneath the urethra. In 1942, Aldridge incorporated the use of rectus fascia and used a separate vaginal incision to incorporate the rectus fascia sling. In addition to muscle and rectus fascia, inorganic materials also have been used for sling grafts. Suburethral slings have been modified by changing the sling material and the anchoring point of the sling. Even with modifications, however, slings basically adhere to the principle of supporting the proximal urethra or bladder neck in a hammock-like fashion, providing a backboard against increases in abdominal pressure.

In 1995, Petros and Ulmsten[2,3] reported on a new ambulatory surgical procedure for the treatment of genuine stress incontinence. The procedure eventually evolved into the tension-free vaginal tape (TVT) procedure. This procedure attempts to recreate urethral support at the level of the pubourethral ligaments by placing a polypropylene sling at the midurethra as opposed to the bladder neck. This synthetic sling is not tied or attached to any other structures. The procedure has the proposed advantages of being done under local anesthesia and being an outpatient surgery.

TECHNIQUE
Transvaginal Approach

In the operating room, the patient is placed in the dorsal supine lithotomy position and prepped and draped in the normal, sterile fashion. The authors routinely have given preoperative antibiotics in the form of first-generation cephalosporin, although randomized data to support this approach are lacking. The bladder is drained with a transurethral 16-Fr Foley catheter. The location of the suprapubic stab incisions is marked with a marking pencil. These incisions should be at the level of the pubic symphysis just lateral to the midline. Placing these incisions too far laterally brings them in close proximity to the pubic tubercle, which potentially risks injury to the ilioinguinal nerves. The skin is infiltrated with 1% lidocaine with epinephrine. The infiltration is initially submucosal and then continues along the backside of the pubic symphysis. Approximately 10 mL of 1% lidocaine with epinephrine is used on either side.

Hydrodissection of the mid to distal anterior vaginal wall is performed with the same solution (approximately 8–10 mL). A 1-cm incision is made

A version of this article was previously published in the *Atlas of the Urologic Clinics of North America* 12:2.

[a] Division of Urogynecology, Department of Obstetrics and Gynecology, Good Samaritan Hospital, Cincinnati, OH, USA

[b] Female Pelvic Medicine and Reconstructive Surgery Fellowship Program Good Samaritan Hospital, 3219 Clifton Avenue, Suite 100, Cincinnati, OH 45220, USA

[c] Division of Urogynecology, The Christ Hospital, 2123 Auburn Avenue, Suite 307, Cincinnati, OH 45219, USA

[d] Departments of Obstetrics and Gynecology and Urology, University of Cincinnati, 2624 Clifton Avenue, Cincinnati, OH 45221, USA

* Corresponding author. Female Pelvic Medicine and Reconstructive Surgery Fellowship Program Good Samaritan Hospital, 3219 Clifton Avenue, Suite 100, Cincinnati, OH 45220.
E-mail address: Steven_Kleeman@trihealth.com

Urol Clin N Am 38 (2011) 39–45
doi:10.1016/j.ucl.2010.12.006

in the midurethra. It is sometimes helpful to feel the bladder neck with the Foley bulb in place to insure that the incision and subsequent placement of the sling is in the midurethra. Allis clamps are placed on the lateral edges of the incision, and Mayo or Metzenbaum scissors are used to create tunnels laterally toward the inferior pubic ramus (**Fig. 1**). While creating the tunnels, the scissors should be pointed and dissecting toward the ipsilateral shoulder. The tunnel should be no bigger than the diameter of the scissors. The scissors should not penetrate the urogenital diaphragm, as this area is important for fixation of the Prolene sling. Because the TVT needle is passed blindly through the retropubic space, a clear understanding of retropubic anatomy is important in avoiding injury to important structures.

Fig. 2 demonstrates the anatomy of the retropubic space. The pubic symphysis is oriented at the 12 o'clock position. Under the pubic symphysis, the urethra is visible coming back to the bladder neck. The arcus tendinous fascia pelvis extends from the back of the pubic symphysis to the ischial spine and is the origin of the levator ani muscles. Above this area, the obturator internus muscle, lateral to the pubic symphysis, is seen, and above the arcus, the obturator neurovascular bundle is seen. Approximately 40% of the time, the obturator artery comes from the external iliac vessels, which exit just under the inguinal ligament into the lower limb. The remaining portion of the time, the obturator artery comes from the anterior division of the obturator artery. Another important blood vessel is the inferior epigastric vessel, which

originates from the external iliac and proceeds medially and cephalad toward the rectus abdominus muscles. Muir and colleagues[4] described the relationship of these vessels to a properly placed TVT needle in 10 fresh cadavers. Distances were measured from the needle to the vessel and from the midpubic bone to the vessel (**Table 1**).

The TVT needle and handle are assembled. The authors find it helpful to place a small hemostat in the midline where the two plastic sheaths overlap. This approach allows for orientation of the midline and prevents the plastic sheaths from pulling apart during insertion. Before insertion of the needle, a urethral guide is inserted into the Foley catheter. This guide allow for deviation of the urethra in a direction opposite to that of the needle. The dominant hand is placed on the handle, and the nondominant hand is used to feel and guide the needle. Initially, the needle tip is introduced into the previously created vaginal tunnels. The tip of the needle should come into direct contact with the inferior pubic ramus. Before advancing the needle, the thumb of the nondominant hand is placed near the junction of the handle, and the needle and index finger are placed in the vaginal lumen pressing against the inferior ramus of the pubis. The direction of the needle's tip is toward the ipsilateral shoulder (**Fig. 3**). As the needle is advanced, the tip of the needle can be felt sliding along the undersurface of the inferior pubic ramus. Gentle pressure on the handle that is applied by the thumbs on both hands is used to penetrate the urogenital diaphragm. Generally, as this structure is transversed, there is a popping sensation or

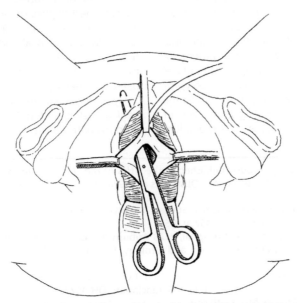

Fig. 1. Allis clamps are placed on the lateral edges of the incision, and Mayo or Metzenbaum scissors are used to create tunnels laterally toward the inferior pubic ramus.

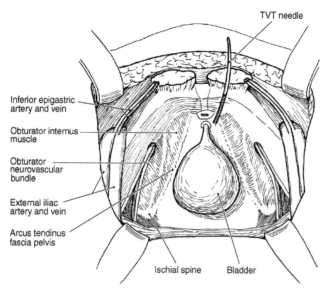

Fig. 2. Anatomy of the retropubic space.

a "giving" feeling. Once the needle is through the urogenital diaphragm, its direction changes, and its tip should be directed toward the previously created suprapubic stab wound on that side. The needle is kept in close proximity to the back of the pubic symphysis while it is advanced through the space of Retsius toward the suprapubic stab wound. It may be difficult to feel the give of the resistance through the urogenital diaphragm. The needle tip should not be advanced more than approximately 2 to 3 cm past the index finger on the undersurface of the inferior pubic ramus before changing the direction of the needle tip to a more medial and superior direction.

The needle should be through the vaginal canal, penetrate the urogenital diaphragm, pass through the space of Retsius, penetrate the rectus muscle and anterior abdominal fascia, and exit from the superior stab wound. With the needle in place, cystourethroscopy is performed. Great care should be taken to look for signs of penetration of the needle into the bladder. Development of hematuria is highly suspicious for a bladder injury.

The bladder well should be distended adequately, and the bladder mucosa should be inspected carefully. The most likely area of bladder injury seems to be the upper lateral area on each side within the dome of the bladder. If no signs of injury are found after thorough inspection of the bladder and urethra, the needle is pulled through, the tape and plastic are cut, and a hemostat is attached to the end of the plastic sleeve. The Foley catheter is reinserted into the bladder. The bladder is drained completely, and the procedure is repeated on the patient's opposite side.

Once the tape has been passed and the needles are removed, tensioning of the tape is performed. The authors generally fill the bladder with 300 mL of sterile water with the cystoscope before tensioning the tape. The tape should be pulled on either side so that the overlapping plastic in the middle of the tape lies underneath the midurethra. If the procedure has been done under local anesthesia with intravenous sedation, the patient is asked to cough. The tape may be tightened and loosened while the patient coughs to find

Table 1
Distance of vessels from TVT needle and midpubic bone (in centimeters)[4]

Vessels	TVT Needle	Midpubic Bone
Superficial epigastric	3.9 (0.9–6.7)	7.2 (4.4–9.3)
Inferior epigastric	3.9 (1.9–6.6)	7.4 (4.8–10.0)
External iliac	4.9 (2.9–6.2)	8.3 (6.5–10.9)
Obturator	3.2 (1.6–4.3)	6.9 (5.2–8.4)

All vessels are lateral to the appropriate placement of the needle. Lateral and cephalad migration of the needle brings it in close proximity to important vascular structures. Mean and range of distances are listed.

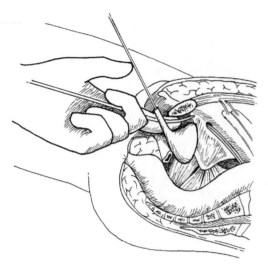

Fig. 3. The needle's tip is directed toward the ipsilateral shoulder. As the needle is advanced, the tip of the needle can be felt sliding along the undersurface of the inferior pubic ramus.

appropriate tensioning. The authors generally like to tension the tape so that there is minimal leakage of urine with forcible coughing. If the procedure is done under general anesthesia, the authors substitute the cough with a Crede maneuver (**Fig. 4**). Repeated downward pressure with

a closed fist in a quick motion in the suprapubic area is used to adjust the tensioning of the tape. Small movements of the tape significantly can alter urethral resistance. Once it is determined that the positioning of the tape is satisfactory, a right-angle clamp is used to hold the tape in the correct position while the plastic sheaths are removed from either side of the tape. Once the plastic sheaths are removed, attempts at moving the tape usually results in only stretching of the tape. After the plastic sheaths are removed, the tape is cut at the surface of the abdominal skin, and the abdominal wound is repaired with a 4.0 absorbable suture. The vaginal mucosa is closed with a 3.0 absorbable suture. A Foley catheter is placed, and a voiding trial is done once the patient can ambulate comfortably to the bathroom.

Suprapubic Approach

The initial infiltration and dissection are the same as outlined in the transvaginal approach; however, the vaginal tunnels should be large enough to permit the tip of an index finger to enter the inferior pubic ramus. The bladder is drained completely, and a urethral guide is placed in the Foley catheter. The surgeon usually grasps the needle with the dominant hand on the handle and the nondominant hand holding on near the tip of the needle (**Fig. 5**).

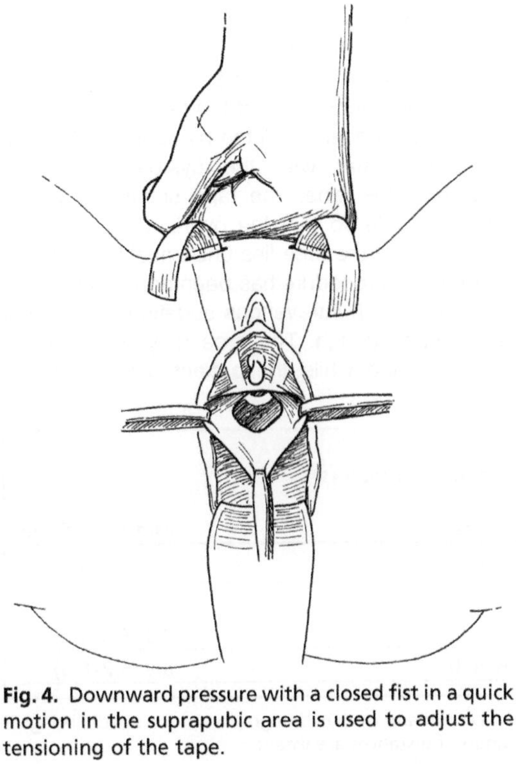

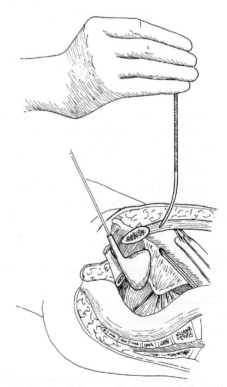

Fig. 4. Downward pressure with a closed fist in a quick motion in the suprapubic area is used to adjust the tensioning of the tape.

Fig. 5. The tip of the needle is inserted through the suprapubic stab wound.

The tip of the needle is inserted through the suprapubic stab wound. Downward pressure is applied by the dominant hand, and the nondominant hand guides the needle off the back of the pubic symphysis (a "giving" sensation or a pop usually is felt as the needle transverses the rectus abdominus fascia). The nondominant hand is removed from the needle, and the index finger of the nondominant hand is placed into the vaginal tunnel on the ipisilateral side of the needle. The dominant hand takes the needle, and the handle is directed toward the abdomen of the patient. The needle is advanced along the back of the pubic symphysis until the tip of the needle is palpated by the index finger of the nondominant hand (**Fig. 6**). The needle exits the vagina at the level of the mid-urethra. Once the tip of the needle is felt by the index finger, continued pressure by the dominant hand on the handle allows the needle to pass through the urogenital diaphragm, and the index finger simultaneously guides the needle out through the vaginal tunnel. The needle is left in place, and the same procedure is repeated on the opposite side. After both needles are in place, cystourethroscopy is done to insure no inadvertent injuries to the bladder. The bladder should be distended fully, and all aspects of the bladder mucosa and urethra should be inspected. Once it is determined that there is no inadvertent injury to the bladder, the TVT needles are attached to the abdominal guide needles by a plastic connector. The polypropylene tape is passed through to the abdomen by gently pushing on the TVT needle

and gently pulling on the transabdominal needle. Once the TVT needle is through the abdominal stab wound, the tape and plastic are cut and tagged with a hemostat. The tensioning procedure is similar to that for the transvaginal approach. Once the appropriate tensioning is done, the plastic sheaths are removed, and the polypropylene tape is cut off at the abdominal skin. The abdominal wounds generally are closed with a 4.0 absorbable suture, and the vaginal incision is closed with a 3.0 absorbable suture.

COMPLICATIONS

The largest series on complication has been the Austrian Registry, which included 2795 patients.[5] Of these patients, 2022 had not undergone surgery for incontinence or pelvic organ prolapse. The bladder perforation rate was 2.7% and was higher in patients who had underwent previous surgery for pelvic organ prolapse or who had incontinence. Intraoperative bleeding was found in 2.3% of the cases, and this rate was similar to the rate in women who had and had not undergone previous surgery. The rate of postoperative urinary tract infections was 17%. A total of 74 patients required reoperation during the postoperative period. Nineteen of these patients underwent surgery for hematoma formation. A total of 68 patients underwent reoperation for voiding dysfunction. One small bowel injury occurred. Karram and colleagues[6] published their complication rates on their first 350 patients of which 20% had undergone previous vaginal or retropubic procedures for stress incontinence. Bladder perforations occurred in 4.9% of patients. Seventeen patients (4.9%) had voiding dysfunction, of which six patients ultimately had the tape cut. Two of these patients developed recurrent stress urinary incontinence. Thirty-eight patients (10.9%) developed at least two urinary tract infections during the postoperative period. Forty-two patients (12%) had persistent urgency and urge incontinence that required anticholinergic therapy for more than 6 weeks after the surgery. One patient developed ilioinguinal nerve injury, one patient developed femoral nerve strain, and another patient developed obturator nerve irritation. All nerve injuries resolved within the first 6 weeks after surgery. Two patients experienced extrusion of the tape or poor healing of the vagina. In one patient, the eroded edge was trimmed, and the vagina advanced. One patient had a breakdown of her incision and was treated with local estrogen cream. One patient had a urethral erosion of the tape; however, this complication developed after repeated urethral

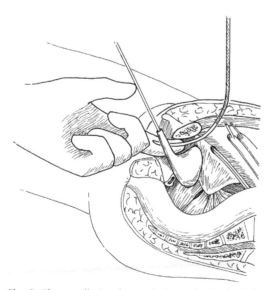

Fig. 6. The needle is advanced along the back of the pubic symphysis until the tip of the needle is palpated by the index finger of the nondominant hand.

dilatations for voiding dysfunction.[7] This patient required excision of the tape and closure of urethrotomy and subsequently redeveloped stress urinary incontinence.

Debodinance[8] reported a 3-year study of 256 TVT procedures. The investigators reported bladder perforation in 5.5% of cases, hematomas in 0.4%, urinary tract infections in 3.1%, urethral injuries in 0.4%, transient urine retention in 5.1%, and de novo urinary urgency in 12%. Several case reports have demonstrated bowel perforation using TVT slings.

RESULTS

Results for the TVT procedure have been encouraging. **Table 2** describes nine studies involving patients who were treated with the TVT procedure. Studies vary by the number of patients; the length of follow-up; and whether patients had preexisting urgency, frequency, or intrinsic sphincter deficiency. In general, cure and improvement rates were lowest for patients who were treated with intrinsic sphincter deficiency and ranged from 86% to 99% for patients with primary stress

Table 2
Studies of the TVT procedure

Author	No. of Patients/ Condition	Length of Follow-up	Type of Testing	Outcome
Wang[9]	39/GSI	Range, 12–24 mo; median, 19 mo	Urodynamics, 1-h pad test	90% of patients cured or improved 10% failed
Olssen and Kroon[10]	51/GSI	36 mo	QOL, 48-h pad test	90% cured 3% improved 4% failed
Gordon et al[11]	30/occult stress incontinence	Mean, 14.25 mo	Urodynamics	No symptomatic SUI 49 patients with persistent DI after surgery 90% cured
Nilsson et al[12]	85/SUI	5 y	URO, QOL, 24-h pad test	84.7% cured 4.7% improved 11 of 25 patients with persistent urge symptoms
Haab et al[13]	62/SUI	Median, 16.2 mo	Questionnaire, stress test	87.1% cured 9% improved 3.3% failed 6.4% with new-onset DI
Rezapour et al[14]	49/GSI and ISD	Mean, 4 y	URO, QOL, pad test	74% cured 12% improved 14% failed
Rezapour[15]	34/recurrent SUI	Mean, 4 y	URO, QOL, 24-h pad test	82% cured 9% improved 9% failed
Ulmsten[16]	131	>12 mo	Stress test, QOL, 24-h pad test, URO	91% cured 9% improved 2% failed
Nilsson[17]	161/GSI	16 mo	URO, stress test, 24-h pad test	94% completely or significantly improved 31% developed de novo urge
Meschia[18]	404	Median, 21 mo	Stress test, URO	92% cured (subjective) 90% cured (objective) 4% improved

Abbreviations: DI, detrusor instability; GSI, genuine stress infection; ISD, intrinsic sphincter deficiency; QOL, quality of life; SUI, stress urinary incontinence.

urinary incontinence. The authors retrospectively examined 151 patients who had filled out pre- and postoperative quality-of-life forms. With a mean follow-up of 22.1 months, there were significant improvements in the postoperative scores for the IIQ-7 (Incontinence Impact Questionnaire) and UDI-6 (Urinary Distress Inventory). Subscales measuring urge symptoms, stress incontinence symptoms, and symptoms of voiding dysfunction showed significant improvement. The improvements were consistent regardless of the type or severity of stress incontinence.[19]

REFERENCES

1. Hofenfellner R, Petrie E. Sling procedures in surgery. In: Stanton SL, Tanagho E, editors. Surgery of female incontinence, 2nd edition. Berlin: Springer-Verlag; 1986. p. 105–13.

2. Petros P, Ulmsten U. Intervaginal slingplasty—an ambulatory surgical procedure for treatment of female stress incontinence. Scand J Urol Nephrol 1995;29:75–82.

3. Ulmsten U, Henriksen L, Johnson P, et al. An ambulatory surgical procedure for treatment of female urinary incontinence. Int Urogynecol J 1996;7:81–6.

4. Muir TW, Tulikangas PK, Paraiso MF, et al. The relationship of tension-free vaginal tape insertion and vascular anatomy. Obstet Gynecol 2003;101(5 Pt 1):933–6.

5. Tamusino KF, Hanzal E, Kolle D, et al. Austrian Urogynecology Working Group—Tension-free vaginal tape operation: results of the Austrian Registry. Obstet Gynecol 2001;98:732–6.

6. Karram MM, Segal JL, Vassallo BJ, et al. Complication and untoward effects of the tension-free vaginal tape procedure. Obstet Gynecol 2003;24:208–11.

7. Vassallo BJ, Kleeman SD, Segal JL, et al. Urethral erosion of a tension-free vaginal tape. Obstet Gynecol 2003;101(5 Pt 2):1055–8.

8. Debodinance. Delporte, Engrand, Boulogne: Tension-free-vaginal tape (TVT) in the treatment of urinary stress incontinence: 3 years experience involving 256 operations. Eur J Obstet Gynecol 2002;105:49–58.

9. Wang AC. An assessment of the early surgical outcome and urodynamic effects of the tension-free vaginal tape (TVT). Int Urogynecol J 2000;11:282–4.

10. Olsson I, Kroon UB. A three-year postoperative evaluation of tension-free vaginal tape. Gynecl Obstet Invest 1999;48:267–9.

11. Gordon D, Gold RS, Pauzner D, et al. Combined genitourinary prolapse repair and prophylactic tension-free vaginal tape in women with severe prolapse and occult stress urinary incontinence: preliminary results. Urology 2001;58:547–50.

12. Nilsson CG, Kuuva N, Falconer C, et al. Long-term results of the tension-free vaginal tape (TVT) procedure for surgical treatment of female stress urinary incontinence. Int Urogynecol J Pelvic Floor Dysfunct 2001;12(Suppl 2):S5–8.

13. Haab F, Sananes S, Amarenco G, et al. Results of the tension-free vaginal tape procedure for the treatment of type II stress urinary incontinence at a minimum follow up of 1 year. J Urol 2001;165:159–62.

14. Rezapour M, Falconer C, Ulmsten U. Tension-free vaginal tape (TVT) in stress incontinent women with intrinsic sphincter deficiency (ISD)—a long term follow-up. Int Urogynecol J Pelvic Floor Dysfunct 2001;12(Suppl 2):S12–4.

15. Rezapour M, Ulmsten U. Tension-free vaginal tape (TVT) in women with recurrent stress urinary incontinence—a long-term follow up. Int Urogynecol J Pelvic Floor Dyfunct 2001;12(Suppl 2):S9–11.

16. Ulmsten U, Falconer C, Johnson P, et al. A multicenter study of tension-free vaginal tape (TVT) for surgical treatment of stress urinary incontinence. Int Urogynecol J 1998;9:210–3.

17. Nilsson CG, Kuuva N. The tension-free vaginal tape procedure is successful in the majority of women with indications for surgical treatment of urinary stress incontinence. Br J Obstet Gynaecol 2001;108:414–9.

18. Meschia M, Pifarotti P, Bernasconi F, et al. Tension-free vaginal tape: analysis of outcomes and complications in 404 stress incontinent women. Int Urogynecol J Pelvic Floor Dysfunct 2001;12-(Suppl 2):S24–7.

19. Vassallo BJ, Kleeman SD, Segal JL, et al. Tension free vaginal tape: a quality-of-life assessment. Obstet Gynecol 2002;100:518–24.

Cystocele Repair with Interpositional Grafting

Patrick B. Leu, MD[a], Harriette M. Scarpero, MD[b],
Roger R. Dmochowski, MD[c],*

KEYWORDS

- Interposition grafting
- Anterior compartment vaginal prolapsed
- Porcine dermis interposition graft

Anterior compartment vaginal prolapse, also known as cystocele, is one of numerous types of pelvic floor relaxation that arise from weakening of the endopelvic fascia and herniation of pelvic viscera through the potential space of the vagina. Weakness of the levator fascia results in loss of pelvic floor support and subsequent formation of anterior compartment defects (the preferable term, according to International Continence Society terminology)[1] or cystoceles.

The fascia of the levator floor serves primarily as a supportive role for the anterior vaginal wall and the bladder and urethra in composite. The abdominal aspect of this fascia is referred to as the endopelvic fascia. The vaginal side is referred to as the perivesical fascia at the level of the bladder base and the periurethral fascia at the level of the bladder neck. The pubocervical fascia is the combined periurethral and perivesical fascia complex. The vaginal and abdominal components of these fascial sheets fuse laterally at their insertion into the tendinous arch of the obturator internus (arcus tendineus fasciae pelvis), which forms the pelvic side wall anchor for these structures.

When viewing vaginal support from cephalad to caudad, the cardinal ligaments support the upper vagina and cervix and anchor them to the pelvic sidewall. In the midvagina, the vesicopelvic ligament extends from the pelvic sidewall to the bladder base and supports it and the anterior vaginal wall. The urethropelvic ligaments support the urethra from the meatus to the bladder neck. The arcuate line (arcus tendineus) of the pelvis, which is the condensation of the obturator internus fascia and endopelvic fascia, provides the lateral support insertion for all of these structures. This strong insertion provides a stabilization point for the entire pelvic floor hammock.[2]

Cystocele defects commonly are associated with other forms of pelvic relaxation, including loss of support of the uterus (uterine descensus), vaginal apex (vault prolapse), and posterior compartment (rectocele). After hysterectomy, enteroceles can occur at the apex of the vaginal vault.

Defects of the anterior compartment may result in isolated defects in urethral support, bladder support, or both. Loss of urethral support may result in urethral hypermobility without a concomitant cystocele defect. Cystoceles are more complex and may involve central defects, lateral defects, or both. Lateral defect cystoceles result from disruption or separation of the condensation of the vesicopelvic ligament to the arcus tendineous on either side of the vagina. Central defect cystoceles result from attenuation of the perivesical (pubocervical) fascia without compromise of the urethropelvic and vesicopelvic ligaments. Central defect cystoceles often are associated with attenuation of upper vaginal support, including loss of

A version of this article was previously published in the *Atlas of the Urologic Clinics of North America* 12:2.
a The Urology Center, P.C., 111 South 90th Street, Omaha, NE 68114, USA
b Associated Urologists, 4230 Harding Road, Suite 521, Nashville, TN 37205, USA
c Department of Urologic Surgery, Vanderbilt University Medical Center, Room A 1302, Medical Center North, Nashville, TN 37232, USA
* Corresponding author.
E-mail address: roger.dmochowski@vanderbilt.edu

cardinal ligament support (with a concomitant enterocele). The most common form of cystocele is a combination cystocele. Isolated central defects comprise less than 10% of diagnosed cystoceles. Isolated lateral defects are more common and often are associated with urethral hypermobility. When central and lateral defects are present, more severe degrees of prolapse often result.

DIAGNOSIS

Diagnosis of anterior compartment defects is made using a complete history and physical examination. A variety of symptoms, such as the sensation of a vaginal mass or bulge, urinary incontinence (stress or urge), urgency, obstruction, dyspareunia, vaginal irritation, and defecatory symptoms, especially with concomitant posterior compartment defects (ie, rectocele), may be present. Physical examination of the vagina demonstrates a mass occupying the anterior vaginal wall from the vaginal apex (or the cervix if a hysterectomy has not been performed) to the bladder neck or urethra. Multichannel videourodynamics is often useful in preoperative evaluation and counseling.

INDICATIONS FOR SURGERY

Symptoms arising from the cystocele and the presence of urinary incontinence form the cornerstone indications for repair. The appropriate operation is based on the degree and severity of the patient's incontinence, magnitude of the cystocele (grade), underlying nature of the fascial defect (central/lateral), and patient's ability to empty the bladder. Comprehensive surgical planning also includes identification of associated prolapse elements (and their symptoms), including enterocele, rectocele, and apical prolapse defects.

The type of anterior compartment repair is indicated by the preoperatively defined fascial defect. Central fascial defects may be managed with a placation type of repair or an interposition graft repair with or without concomitant sling, and the choice depends on the presence of incontinence. Isolated central defect repair is rare in the absence of a concomitant stress incontinence procedure.

Lateral defect repairs may be performed with a variety of techniques, including multiple-point repairs (four- or six-corner bladder suspensions) and vaginal–paravaginal or abdominal–paravaginal repairs with combined incontinence intervention. Severe cystoceles with combined central and lateral defects require concomitant stress procedures and interpositional graft placement to compensate for complete disruption of the supportive pelvic floor structures.

Surgical Technique

The patient is placed in the dorsal lithotomy position with the aid of hydraulic stirrups. No extremity is flexed greater than 90°. After prepping the abdomen, perineum, and vagina, the posterior compartment is draped away from the surgical field. Access under an adherent drape is still possible, if necessary. A weighted speculum and a ring retractor are used for vaginal exposure.

A Foley catheter is placed, and hydrodissection of the anterior vaginal wall is performed with normal saline or dilute vasoconstrictor. Dissection begins with a midline incision from the midurethra to vaginal apex (**Fig. 1**). The anterior vaginal wall, overlying the cystocele, is dissected away from the underlying attenuated pubocervical fascia (**Fig. 2**). The dissection plane is identified by the glistening white pubocervical fascia, and the vaginal wall is thin in this plane. Dissection in the wrong plane usually is associated with significant bleeding and inability to identify the underlying fascia.

Once dissection of the vaginal wall has been completed to the fornix on either side of the bladder neck, sharp dissection is used to penetrate the endopelvic fascia and enter the retropubic space immediately under the arch of the pubis (**Fig. 3**). This plane is generally avascular and should separate easily from the underlying fascial components. In cases that previously underwent surgery, this space may be difficult to identify, and sharp, shallow dissection (immediate proximity to the arch of the symphysis pubis) should be used to avoid inadvertent entry into the pelvic viscera, including the bladder and urethra.

After entry into the retropubic space, lateral dissection of the endopelvic fascia from the urethra to the bladder base is performed to mobilize these structures (**Fig. 4**). Subsequently, dissection is performed to the vaginal cuff in a line parallel to the orientation of the vaginal vault. In women who have undergone a hysterectomy, the stump of the uterine arterial complex commonly is encountered during this dissection, and bleeding may occur as a result of disruption of this structure. Suture ligature of these vessels with 4-0 polydioxanone should be contemplated to avoid persistent blood loss during the reconstructive segment of the operation. Cautery should be minimized to avoid devascularization of the underlying tissues.

Apical dissection should be meticulous to aid in identifying any enterocele component; if found, the

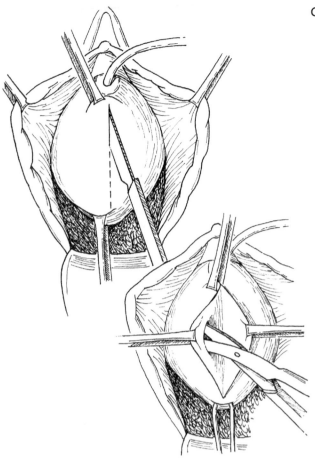

Fig. 1. A midline incision on the anterior vaginal wall is made from the midurethra to the apex of the vaginal vault.

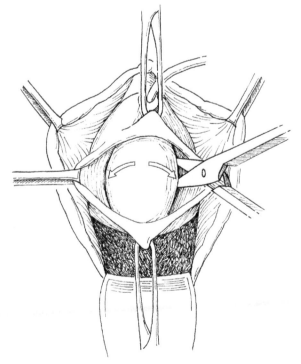

Fig. 2. Dissection of the vaginal wall away from the underlying pubocervical fascia is performed bilaterally and posteriorly.

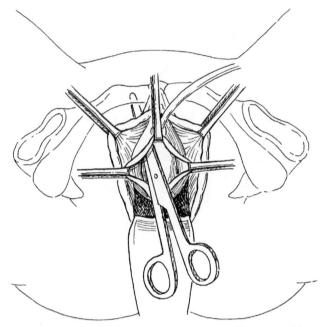

Fig. 3. The endopelvic fascia is penetrated sharply to allow entry into the retropubic space.

defect should be excised and closed. Apical enteroceles may be small and somewhat obscured by the bladder base descensus. The cardinal ligaments often can be identified at this level of the dissection; and when they are found, plication with a 0 or 2-0 synthetic absorbable suture (SAS) can be performed. If there is significant apical descensus, posterior placement of sutures in the coccygeus region provides further support and stability to the anterior compartment repair. Number one polydiaxonone suture (PDS) sutures

are placed 1 cm inferior and medial to the ischial spines through the iliococcygeus muscle (**Fig. 5**). Great care must be taken to place these sutures as described to avoid injury to the pudendal neurovasculature and ureter, which are in close proximity. These vault suspension sutures are brought through the vaginal apex to be tied at the completion of the procedure, after the vaginal wall has been closed.

Once dissection of the retropubic space is completed and the space is freely mobile, a sling is placed. The sling may be made of autologous tissue harvested through a separate abdominal incision or made of any of a variety of tissues, including autograft, allograft, xenograft, or synthetic. Ligature passage needles are directed from suprapubic to vaginal incisions on either side of proximal urethra and bladder neck using digital guidance. Once placed, cystoscopy is performed to exclude needle entry into the bladder or urethra. Suspending 0 or 1 polypropylene sutures or SASs are placed through either end of the sling material, and the suspending suture is transposed from vaginal to suprapubic incisions using the ligature carrier. The sling is affixed to the underlying periurethral fascia with 4-0 SAS.

After these steps are completed, a 0 or 2-0 absorbable or nonabsorbable suture is placed in the obturator internus fascia at the level of the arcuate line in an interrupted manner from bladder neck to vaginal apex. This step usually requires the use of two to four sutures in sequence.

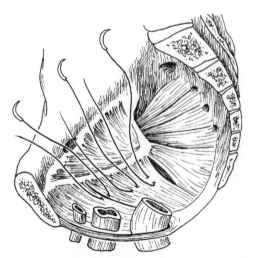

Fig. 4. Further lateral dissection of the endopelvic fascia allows mobilization of the bladder and urethra.

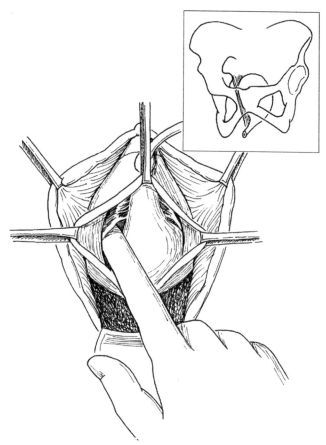

Fig. 5. Vault suspension sutures are placed 1 cm medial and distal to the ischial spines.

A sheet of graft material measuring 6 × 8 cm or 8 × 8 cm (depending on the dimensions of the defect) is affixed to the preplaced sutures (**Fig. 6**). The material should be placed loosely under the bladder base from the bladder neck to vaginal apex. A suture also is placed at the vaginal apex (**Fig. 7**). This step incorporates the cardinal ligament complex and further supports the posterior aspect of the repair. Excess vaginal wall tissue is excised, and the vaginal wall is closed with a running 2-0 SAS. Vaginal vault suspension sutures (if placed) are tied at this juncture.

After completion of the previous steps, cystoscopy again is performed to ensure that no penetration of the bladder has occurred, there is bilateral efflux from both ureteral orifices, and the bladder base has been corrected with the inlay material. Sling tension is set, and the suprapubic incision is closed.

A vaginal pack is placed. Twelve to 24 hours after the operation, the pack is removed, and the patient performs a voiding trial. If this trial is not successful, the Foley catheter is reinserted, or intermittent catheterization may begin. Alternatively, if a suprapubic tube has been placed at the time of surgery, the patient can cycle the suprapubic tube at home. Lifting of objects greater than 5 lb is avoided for 6 weeks.

OUTCOMES
Complications

Intraoperative complications with this procedure are rare. They include injury to associated structures, such as the urethra, bladder, and ureters. Bleeding and infection are rarely problematic. Familiarity with the anatomy of the female pelvis and attention to surgical technique and fundamentals help minimize the incidence of complications. Intraoperative cystoscopic evaluation, with the aid of intravenous indigo carmine, confirms the integrity of the bladder and patency of the ureters.

Postoperative voiding dysfunction rarely is seen and should be discussed preoperatively. Frequently, an element of this complication is present before the surgery, and this fact supports

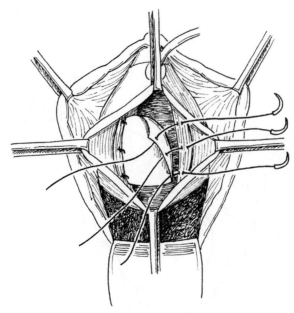

Fig. 6. After sling placement, absorbable sutures are placed in the obturator internus fascia on either side, from the bladder neck to vaginal apex. The sutures are passed through their corresponding position in the graft and secured.

the role of urodynamic testing as part of the initial evaluation.

Results

The authors reviewed the results of 70 patients with high-grade cystocele (grades III–IV) who underwent repair with porcine dermis interposition graft.

Patients underwent preoperative multichannel videourodynamics. Sixty-five patients underwent concomitant pubovaginal sling, and 50 patients also had vault suspension performed. Average follow-up was 24 months. No intraoperative complications occurred. Fifty-nine patients (91%) were dry. One patient had a recurrence of vault prolapse without cystocele, which was corrected

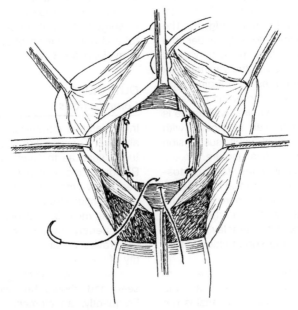

Fig. 7. A suture that is placed at the vaginal apex incorporates the cardinal ligament complex.

with abdominal sacralcolpopexy. Six patients (8.6%) experienced recurrence of grade II cystocele, but were asymptomatic. Three patients (4.3%) demonstrated recurrent grade III cystocele but elected no further intervention. Six patients (8.6%) developed de novo low-grade rectoceles. One superficial vaginal wound separation was treated conservatively.

SUMMARY

A systematic approach to the repair of cystoceles using interposition grafting is discussed. Surgeons' opinions vary regarding which graft material is most appropriate. The choices for mesh interposition include synthetic, xenograft, autograft (free full thickness vaginal wall), and allograft materials. Long-term data are not available to support the use of one material over another; however, an abundance of literature has documented results of different materials used in urethral sling surgery, and these data are important to consider. Although a review of biomaterial selection is beyond the scope of this article, the authors favor porcine dermis xenografts.

Defect repair may be addressed with a single-component interposition graft, which serves as a bladder base and urethral support,[3] or with a two-component interposition using different grafts for the sling and the anterior compartment repair. The authors favor the latter approach.

High-grade cystocele repair using the porcine dermis interposition graft is successful and associated with few complications. Cystocele recurrence is typically low grade and does not require additional surgery.

REFERENCES

1. Bump RC, Mattiasson A, Bo K, et al. The standardization of terminology of pelvic organ prolapse and pelvic floor dysfunction. Am J Obstet Gyneol 1996; 175:10–7.
2. Delancey JOL. Anatomic aspects of vaginal eversion after hysterectomy. Am J Obstet Gynecol 1992;166: 1717–28.
3. Kobashi KC, Mee SL, Leach GE. A new technique for cystocele repair and transvaginal sling: the cadaveric prolapse repair and sling (CAPS). Urology 2000;56:9–14.

Female Urethral Reconstruction

Nirit Rosenblum, MD*, Victor W. Nitti, MD

KEYWORDS

- Proximal and bladder neck • Midurethra • Distal urethra

The female urethra is relatively short compared with its male counterpart and is generally between 2 and 4 cm in length. It is made up of an inner layer of mucosal epithelium with numerous infoldings that create an effective seal against the passive loss of urine. Beneath the mucosa lies a rich, vascular network of elastic tissue that is much like the corpus spongiosum. Surrounding the spongy vascular tube is a collagen-rich fibromuscular envelope comprising the periurethral fascia. These three components of a normal urethra are crucial in maintaining continence and enabling dynamic function during increases in abdominal pressure and during normal micturition.

Two fascial attachments suport the urethra: the pubourethral and urethropelvic ligaments. The pubourethral ligaments are a band of fascial support located superiorly between the urethra and pubic symphysis. These ligaments often serve as a point of anatomic division between the proximal and distal urethra. The urethropelvic ligaments are comprised of two layers of fascial condensation, the endopelvic fascia and the pubocervical fascia, which provide lateral attachment to the arcus tendineus. The midurethra is believed to be the center of continence where the striated sphincter complex maintains active and passive tone.

A basic understanding of female urethral anatomy is necessary to approach urethral reconstruction from an anatomic standpoint. This article reviews the techniques of female urethral reconstruction based on these anatomic divisions: proximal and bladder neck, midurethra, and distal urethra.

BLADDER NECK AND PROXIMAL URETHRA

The bladder neck and proximal urethra are made up primarily of smooth muscle that is oriented in a circular fashion. This intrinsic, involuntary sphincter maintains passive continence in addition to the striated urethral sphincter. Failure of the bladder neck sphincteric mechanism can be related to age, childbirth, neurologic disease, congenital anomalies, and pelvic surgery. Intrinsic sphincter deficiency is a common finding in women with stress incontinence and is apparent as funneling of the bladder neck during the filling phase on cystography. Reconstruction of the bladder neck to restore continence can be accomplished in several ways depending on the severity of incontinence, its underlying cause and associated anatomic defects, and the goals of surgical correction. This article describes the technical aspects of bladder neck reconstruction in women, specifically pubovaginal sling placement, surgical closure of the bladder neck, and placement of an artificial urinary sphincter.

Pubovaginal Sling

Traditionally, pubovaginal sling surgery has been used to treat intrinsic sphincter deficiency and stress urinary incontinence, with concomitant correction of hypermobility and restoration of posterior urethral support. Sling materials include autologous fascia, allografts, xenografts, and synthetics.[1] The most common pubovaginal sling technique involves harvesting a strip of autologous fascia, generally rectus abdominis fascia or fascia

A version of this article was previously published in the *Atlas of the Urologic Clinics of North America* 12:2.
Department of Urology, New York University, Langone Medical Center, 150 East 32 Street, New York, NY 10016, USA
* Corresponding author.
E-mail address: Nirit.Rosenblum@nyumc.org

Urol Clin N Am 38 (2011) 55–64
doi:10.1016/j.ucl.2010.12.008

lata, which is fashioned as a 2 cm × 10- to 15-cm strip. This technique is considered the gold-standard surgical treatment of genuine stress urinary incontinence.

With the patient in the dorsolithotomy position, an incision is made in the anterior vaginal wall at the level of the bladder neck, identifiable by palpation of a Foley catheter balloon. A submucosal tunnel is created beneath the bladder neck and is extended to the endopelvic fascia laterally, which subsequently is perforated to accommodate passage of the sling into the retropubic space. The autologous fascial sling is prepared by passage of nonabsorbable suture through either end. After closure of the fascial harvest site, the sling is placed beneath the bladder neck and passed into the retropubic space above the rectus abdominis fascia. Passage of the sling sutures into the retropubic space can be accomplished using a double-pronged passer (such as the Raz-Peyrera) or a long clamp under finger guidance, taking care to avoid medial deviation. The bladder should be relatively nondistended to avoid inadvertent cystotomy. A cystoscopy should be performed after sling suture passage to ensure bladder integrity and to assess for the presence of any suture material within the bladder lumen. The sling sutures are tied loosely in the midline, above the rectus abdominis fascia, to avoid excessive tension on the bladder neck. A Foley catheter is left in place after surgery until normal voiding ensues, generally between several days to several weeks.

Modifications to this technique include the use of bone anchors for sling fixation, various materials for sling preparation (ie, allograft, xenograft, synthetics), and in situ suspension of the vaginal wall sling. Numerous modifications to the traditional autologous sling technique have been devised to reduce the morbidity associated with autologous fascial harvest. The specifics of these modifications are discussed elsewhere in this issue.

Closure of the Transvaginal Bladder Neck

Surgical closure of the bladder neck in females is indicated in cases of extensive urethral destruction, usually because of a chronic indwelling urethral catheter in cases of neurogenic bladder. Progressive urethral dilatation leads to chronic, intractable incontinence around an indwelling catheter, with associated perineal excoriation and chronic urinary tract infection. Bladder neck closure can be readily accomplished using a transvaginal approach, thereby obviating the need for a complete urinary diversion or transabdominal closure. The bladder then can be managed with an indwelling suprapubic catheter unless a catheterizable stoma is desirable. This technique is analogous to perineal closure of the male urethra for refractory incontinence.

Transvaginal bladder neck closure is accomplished in the dorsolithotomy position. Initially, the surgeon can place a suprapubic cystotomy unless another form of bladder drainage has been established, such as a continent stoma (ie, Mitrofanoff) or an incontinent stoma (ie, ileal bladder chimney). A simple, percutaneous suprapubic cystotomy can be performed using a curved Lowsley retractor or by open technique if indicated.[2] Slight traction on the suprapubic catheter prevents bleeding from the cystotomy and extravasation of urine into the retropubic space.

The anterior vaginal wall is incised, circumscribing the damaged urethra and extending onto the anterior vaginal wall in an inverted U-shaped configuration (**Fig. 1**). This approach allows the creation of an anterior vaginal wall flap by dissection from the underlying perivesical and periurethral fascia. Dissection of the bladder neck is extended laterally to the endopelvic fascia and pubic rami. The endopelvic fascia is perforated sharply to allow adequate mobilization of the bladder neck and base (**Fig. 2**). Indigo carmine is administered intravenously to allow cystoscopic visualization of the ureteral orifices and their proximity to the bladder neck.

The remaining damaged urethra is excised completely, and closure of the bladder neck is

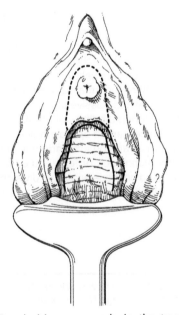

Fig. 1. Two incisions are made in the transvaginal approach to bladder neck closure: One circumscribes the damaged urethra, and the other is an inverted U-shaped flap of anterior vaginal wall epithelium.

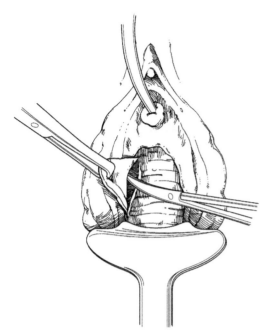

Fig. 2. Dissection of the bladder neck is performed bilaterally to the endopelvic fascia, with perforation into the retropubic space, allowing complete mobilization of the bladder neck and base.

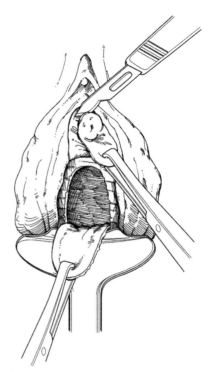

Fig. 3. The damaged urethra is excised in preparation for bladder neck closure.

performed (**Fig. 3**). A running suture of absorbable material is placed in the mucosa, followed by a second layer of suture placed in the perivesical fascia and muscular bladder wall (**Fig. 4**). The second suture line extends from the bladder neck to the anterior bladder wall behind the pubic symphysis, thereby placing the closed bladder neck in the retropubic space. This step avoids direct apposition of suture lines, which may lead to fistula development. The anterior vaginal wall flap is advanced as a third layer (**Fig. 5**).[2] If the vaginal and perivesical tissues are compromised secondary to chronic infection or before radiation therapy, additional tissue interposition can be accomplished by use of a Martius labial fat pad flap. A vaginal pack impregnated with antibiotic cream is left for 24 hours after surgery. The native bladder then can be managed with a chronic, indwelling suprapubic cystotomy or creation of a catheterizable stoma with augmentation cystoplasty in cases of reduced capacity, impaired compliance, or vesicoureteral reflux.

In certain circumstances, it may be desirable to perform bladder neck closure by an abdominal approach. This step can be done transvesically or extravesically.[3]

Artificial Urinary Sphincter

Although commonly used in males with stress urinary incontinence, the artificial urinary sphincter

(AUS) has had limited use in females and generally is reserved for treating extreme cases of incontinence involving multiple failed anti-incontinence operations (type III stress incontinence), neuropathic bladder dysfunction, or congenital anomalies. There have been reports of experience with and outcomes of AUS in female children and adolescents with underlying neuropathic bladder or exstrophy–epispadias complex.[4,5] Long-term continence after AUS placement has been reportedly lower in females than in males, and females have an associated increased risk for AUS explantation.[6] Previous pelvic radiation therapy is a contraindication to AUS placement in females because of the high risks for erosion and device explantation.[7]

AUS placement in females can be performed transabdominally or transvaginally with placement of the cuff at the bladder neck. Broad-spectrum intravenous antibiotics that are targeted at coverage of gram-positive skin flora, gram-negative organisms, and anaerobes are administered on the day of surgery and after surgery. Urine must be sterile before surgery. The avoidance of a urethral catheter before surgery is ideal to minimize infection.[7] Meticulous surgical technique is also necessary to reduce postoperative morbidity.

Transabdominal approach
In women, the retropubic, extraperitoneal approach to AUS placement most commonly is employed.

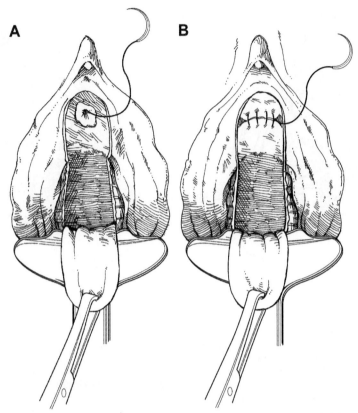

Fig. 4. (*A*) The bladder neck mucosa is closed with a vertical, running suture. (*B*) Bladder wall and perivesical fascia are sutured in a horizontal fashion as a second layer.

The retropubic space generally is entered through a lower abdominal or Pfannenstiel incision, and mobilization of the bladder neck, distal to the ureteral orifices, is performed. Posteriorly, the vesicovaginal plane carefully is dissected just superior to the endopelvic fascia. Any incidental cystotomy or vaginal opening should be sutured in two layers with absorbable suture material to achieve a watertight closure.[8]

The cuff sizer is applied to measure the circumference of the bladder neck, allowing selection of a cuff that is not excessively tight or loose. The cuff is passed carefully around the bladder neck and locked, avoiding the use of sharp instruments in this area. The AUS pump generally is placed within the labia majora, and the balloon reservoir is placed in the preperitoneal rectus abdominis muscle space. The system is cycled after all connections have been made and is left deactivated. A Foley catheter is left in place overnight.[8]

Transvaginal approach

The transvaginal approach to AUS placement in women allows dissection of the urethrovaginal plane under direct visualization. This plane can be obliterated or extensively scarred after previous anti-incontinence procedures, making the transabdominal approach to dissection challenging and resulting in an associated risk for urethral, bladder neck, or vaginal injury.

A vertical incision is made in the anterior vaginal wall from the level of the midurethra to the proximal bladder neck. The vaginal flaps are dissected free laterally toward the endopelvic fascia and should be thick, as they will provide coverage of the AUS. The urethra and bladder neck are freed from their lateral attachments to the pelvic floor musculature and vaginal wall and from their anterior attachments to the pubic symphysis. In cases of extensive scarring, an additional suprameatal incision can be made to allow better access to the anterior surface of the urethra and bladder neck.[9] Ultimately, a circumferential dissection of the bladder neck is accomplished in preparation for cuff placement.

The device is left deactivated at the time of operation, and patients return between 4 and 6 weeks after surgery for AUS activation. Thomas and colleagues[7] reported their experience with 68 female patients undergoing AUS placement. They used a 71- to 80-cm water balloon, except in cases of significant bladder neck scarring, atrophy of

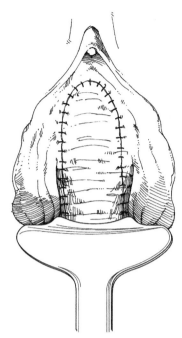

Fig. 5. The anterior vaginal wall flap is advanced and sutured as a third layer of repair.

tissues, or decreased vascularity, in which they used a 61- to 70-cm water balloon.[6] Some investigators advocate the use of a lower-pressure reservoir (51–60 cm of water) in women to prevent device erosion.[9] In general, patients with genuine stress incontinence (type III) alone have a better long-term prognosis with AUS placement and have significantly decreased rates of explantation, whereas patients with neuropathic incontinence exhibit higher rates of infection and device erosion (approximately 50%), requiring explantation.[7] The rates of continence after AUS placement in the neuropathic population remain high (approximately 90%).

MIDURETHRA

The midsegment or proximal segment of the female urethra, between the true bladder neck and pubourethral ligaments, contains the striated sphincter complex and levator ani insertion. The authors believe that the most critical components of active and passive continence are located in this important segment of urethra. Sling surgery for stress incontinence has been targeted at the midurethra rather than the bladder neck, where pubovaginal slings have been placed traditionally. Placement of sling material in the midurethra causes scarring and fixation of the urethra to the pubic bone, thereby recreating the damaged or attenuated pubourethral ligaments. The sling material beneath the urethra reinforces the suburethral vaginal hammock,

protecting against incontinence during increases in abdominal pressure.[1] Intrinsic sphincter deficiency and urethral hypermobility can be treated with a midurethral sling, and this approach has excellent long-term outcomes that are comparable with outcomes for the traditional pubovaginal sling.

Intrinsic damage of the midurethra can lead to stress incontinence, total incontinence, or stricture with resultant obstruction. The treatment of stress and total incontinence is discussed elsewhere in this issue. This discussion focuses on reconstruction of the female midurethra for cases of stricture, sling erosion, and urethrovaginal fistula. Stricture of the female urethra is caused by radiation therapy for pelvic malignancies, previous urethral instrumentation or endoscopic surgery, trauma, iatrogenic injury during urethral diverticulectomy, and gynecologic surgery. Increasing numbers of anti-incontinence surgeries and the widespread use of synthetic sling materials have made urethral erosion a well-recognized morbidity, requiring sling removal and urethral reconstruction. Urethrovaginal fistula related to prolonged childbirth is a common finding in underdeveloped countries, but this complication also can occur after urologic and gynecologic surgery.

Urethral Reconstruction for Stricture

The treatment algorithm for female urethral stricture is not as well defined as the male counterpart. This discrepancy may be attributable to the relative rarity of stricture disease in women, especially in cases of blunt pelvic trauma. Because of the female urethra's short length, anatomic position behind the pubic arch, and relative mobility, the incidence of stricture that occurs after trauma in females is low (range, 0%–6%).[10] More commonly, stricture disease in women is seen after pelvic radiation therapy for gynecologic malignancies and can occur many years later. Generally, repair of stricture disease is divided into endoscopic and open repairs, with the use of local tissue flaps or graft interposition. Because of the relatively short length of the female urethra (approximately 4 cm), stricture excision and end-to-end urethroplasty are not feasible as in male patients.

Endoscopic repair

Midurethral stricture can be treated endoscopically with a cold knife or a Holmium laser. The laser technique requires use of a large-diameter (500–1000 μm) fiber and high-energy and high-frequency settings for effective tissue penetration and cutting. Incisions are performed at the 3 o'clock and 9 o'clock positions with an additional 12 o'clock incision when necessary. A urethral catheter, generally sized 16 Fr or larger, is left in place for several days after surgery. Use of clean intermittent catheterization after surgery can help reduce the risk for recurrence; however, the ideal regimen and duration have not been well defined.

In severe cases of midurethral stricture that are not amenable to simple optical urethrotomy as previously described, a "cut to the light" procedure can be performed.[10] This procedure necessitates placement of a flexible cystoscope in an antegrade fashion to help in the identification of the obliterated urethral segment and the true bladder neck. Such complex cases require prolonged postoperative catheterization to ensure complete healing and re-epithelialization.

Open repair: flap urethroplasty

Vaginal flap urethroplasty can be used to recreate a functional urethra by way of local, healthy tissues. This technique also can improve urethral length in cases of a shortened urethra that is associated with vaginal voiding. A flap of vaginal epithelium in a U-shaped configuration can be employed as a patch or posterior plate of tissue (**Fig. 6**A). A vertical incision in the anterior vaginal wall located directly beneath the urethra allows adequate dissection of the urethra. A longitudinal incision in the posterior urethra is made, effectively exposing the entire segment of strictured or diseased urethra, until more proximal and viable tissue is identified. The vaginal flap is harvested by incising the more cephalad, anterior vaginal wall in a U-shaped configuration, approximately

1.0 to 1.5 cm in width. This flap is flipped up and sutured to the edges of the open posterior urethra using absorbable suture material (**Fig. 6**B).[11] The anterior vaginal wall is closed primarily, creating a second layer of tissue beneath the newly created urethra. In cases of compromised anterior vaginal wall tissue, coverage can be attained by use of labial or local thigh flaps. An additional technique of vaginal flap urethroplasty has been described in which bilateral incisions that are parallel and adjacent to the urethral meatus are used. Vaginal wall flaps are dissected laterally on either side of the urethra and are sutured together in the midline over a 14-Fr urethral catheter (**Figs. 7**A and B).[12]

If extensive scarring or destruction of the anterior vaginal wall is found, local flaps can be used to reconstruct the diseased urethral segment. A rotational flap using labia minora can be harvested to create a neourethra by tubularization over a catheter. In cases of vaginal flap or local flap urethroplasty, additional tissue, such as a Martius labial fat pad graft, can be used to bolster the closure and provide an additional layer of viable tissue.[12] After surgery, a urethral catheter generally is left in place for approximately 1 to 3 weeks, which is when flap urethroplasty is performed.

In patients with preoperative intrinsic sphincteric incompetence, performance of a simultaneous pubovaginal sling procedure can improve postoperative continence. In general, the use of synthetics is not advocated in the setting of urethral reconstruction, and most surgeons use autologous fascia,

A   **B**

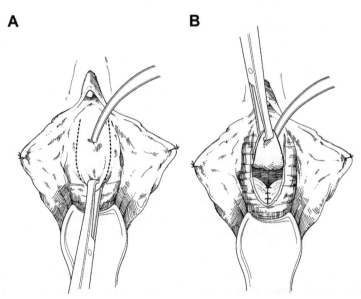

Fig. 6. (*A*) Vaginal flap urethroplasty. A U-shaped incision of the anterior vaginal wall is performed. (*B*) The vaginal wall flap is transposed to the shortened or damaged urethra by tubularization or as a posterior plate of tissue.

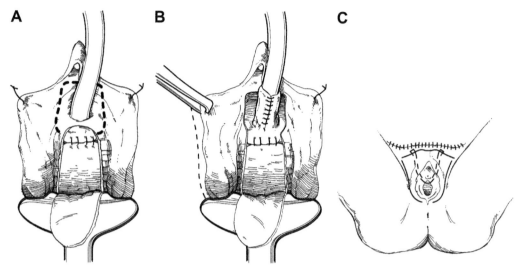

Fig. 7. (*A*) Vaginal wall urethroplasty. Lateral vaginal wall incisions are made parallel to the urethral meatus, with an additional anterior vaginal wall flap (U-shaped configuration). (*B*) The vaginal epithelium is tubularized over a catheter, creating a neourethra. The U-shaped, anterior vaginal wall flap is advanced over the neourethra as an additional layer of tissue. (*C*) A pubovaginal sling of autologous fascia can be placed after creation of the neourethra to provide additional suburethral support.

when available (**Fig. 7**C). Although biologic materials such as allografts or xenografts can be used, little published experience supports this practice; the authors prefer to use autologous fascia for this purpose. The autologous fascial sling is placed over the grafted tissue and the Martius flap, if used. Vaginal packing is used for 24 hours after surgery, and a voiding cystourethrogram is performed to ensure urethral patency and exclude extravasation.[12]

An additional technique for female urethral reconstruction, bladder flap urethroplasty, uses well-vascularized tissue, which heals well without stricture formation. This flap contains circular smooth muscle and α-adrenergic receptors, both of which facilitate continence. These factors are useful for more proximal injuries or complete urethral loss. Hemal and colleagues[13] describe this technique in females with extensive urethral loss secondary to pelvic fracture. An oblique or vertical anterior bladder flap is raised beginning at the level of the bladder neck, and its vascularity is based superolaterally on the dome. Use of the oblique flap avoids placement of a suture line that abuts the anterior vaginal wall suture line, reducing the risk for fistula formation. Vertical bladder flaps provide more length than oblique flaps, which are limited by the location of the ureteral orifice. The flap is tubularized over a catheter. A space between the anterior vaginal wall and pubic bone is created by sharp dissection to allow routing of the neourethra into the vestibule. The neourethra is anastomosed

into position, creating a neomeatus. Concomitantly, bladder neck suspension or pubovaginal sling placement can be performed to improve continence.

Urethral Reconstruction for Sling Erosion

Urethral erosion is defined as entrance of sling material into the urethral lumen and is generally attributable to the use of synthetic materials such as Protegen, Marlex, silicone, and polypropylene. Treatment of urethral erosion includes complete removal of the offending material and reconstruction of the urethra using the techniques previously described, depending on the extent of urethral injury. After complete surgical removal of the foreign body that is causing erosion, the edges of the damaged urethra are debrided carefully, and the defect is closed primarily, if possible. Absorbable suture material of small caliber is used (4-0 or 5-0) on the urethral mucosa. The periurethral fascia must be closed as a separate layer to reduce the risk for fistula formation. In cases of extensive urethral and periurethral damage or inflammation, an interposing Martius flap can be used to provide additional reinforcement of the primary repair. A urethral catheter is left in place after surgery for several days, depending on the extent of urethral repair. If a concomitant sling is indicated for treatment of stress incontinence, an autologous fascial sling is preferable once an adequate urethral repair has been accomplished.[16]

Urethrovaginal Fistula Repair

Preoperative surgical planning by careful vaginal examination is necessary for a successful outcome of urethrovaginal fistula repair. Attention is paid to the extent of urethral tissue loss and the availability of local tissue for reconstruction. Generally, the anterior vaginal wall provides adequate tissue for reconstructive purposes. Alternatively, pedicled labial, perineal, rectus, gracilis, and bladder flaps can be used when anterior vaginal wall tissue seems to be compromised. The principles of fistula repair include adequate exposure of the site; creation of a tension-free, multilayered closure; adequate blood supply to the involved tissues; and adequate bladder drainage.[14] Generally, a large caliber suprapubic cystotomy tube and a urethral catheter are placed for postoperative bladder drainage.

An inverted U-shaped anterior vaginal flap incision is performed just proximal to the fistula site, which will serve as a final layer of tissue overlying the reconstructed urethra. A small fistula usually can be closed primarily with 4-0 or 5-0 absorbable suture material. The mucosal edges are reapproximated, and the adjacent periurethral fascia is closed as a second layer. The anterior vaginal wall flap serves as a third and final layer. The closure can be tested intraoperatively by injection of a methylene blue solution directly into the urethra using a catheter-tipped syringe or a large angiocatheter attached to a 10-mL syringe. Sites of leakage can be sutured directly to provide a watertight closure. In cases of more extensive urethral tissue loss, reconstruction can be accomplished with pedicled, local tissue flaps, as previously described in the section on flap urethroplasty. A Martius flap can provide an additional layer of healthy, vascularized tissue.

In cases of more complex and refractory urethrovaginal fistulas, Bruce and colleagues[15] described the use of a pedicled rectus abdominis muscle flap. These investigators advocate the use of this flap when previous Martius flap interposition has failed, as this procedure is considered the gold-standard flap treatment for urologic and gynecologic reconstruction. This technique involves a combined retropubic and vaginal approach involving multilayered closure of the fistula, as previously described. The left rectus abdominis muscle is harvested from its fascial sheath and tubularized with interrupted, absorbable suture. The inferior epigastric vessels must be preserved. This tube of muscle is passed through the endopelvic fascia and into the vaginal incision and is used as a support for the suburethral and subtrigonal areas, providing extensive tissue coverage of the fistula. The distal end of the muscle is secured to the contralateral arcus tendineus, obturator fascia, or Cooper's ligament. The Foley catheter is left indwelling after surgery for 7 days; most patients require clean intermittent catheterization for a period of time (range, 7–21 days) after

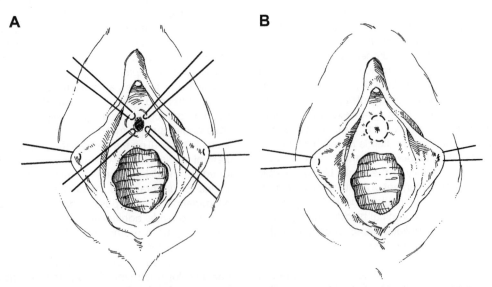

Fig. 8. (*A*) Initially, sutures are placed circumferentially in more proximal, healthy urethral mucosa. (*B*) Circumferential excision of the distal, diseased, or stenotic urethra before performance of advancement meatoplasty.

catheter removal. All six cases described in this study were cured of their refractory urethrovaginal fistulas, and no recurrences occurred at a mean follow-up of 22 months.[15]

DISTAL URETHRA

Stenosis or stricture of the distal urethra in women often presents with lower urinary tract symptoms that are consistent with obstruction. This situation can be seen after traumatic urethral instrumentation and endoscopic procedures, after radiation therapy to the pelvis or vulva for gynecologic malignancy, and more commonly in postmenopausal women with vulvar dystrophy or significant vaginal atrophy from estrogen deficiency. Meatotomy can be performed to treat this distal stenosis by simple incision of the meatus; however, in the authors' experience, circumferential, distal urethrectomy and advancement meatoplasty work best for treating distal strictures and can be applied to any stricture within 5 to 10 mm from the meatus. The technique involves preplacement of interrupted absorbable sutures in the more proximal, healthy urethral mucosa (at least 2 mm proximal to the strictured segement), so that the mucosa does not retract inward (**Fig. 8**A). A circumferential excision of the distal urethra and meatus is performed (**Fig. 8**B). The healthy mucosa is advanced and sutured circumferentially to the vaginal epithelium in an interrupted fashion. In effect, a neomeatus is created with well-vascularized, nondiseased mucosa. Depending on the degree of reconstruction, a urethral catheter can be left in place for 1 to 3 days after surgery. Topical estrogen cream can promote wound healing and improve mucosal function to prevent recurrence of stricture.

SUMMARY

Reconstruction of the female urethra is accomplished by adherence to several basic principles: anatomic considerations with special attention to concomitant incontinence; reconstruction in a multilayered fashion with healthy, well-vascularized tissues; use of local tissue flaps as an additional layer of tissue; and avoidance of the use of synthetic materials in the setting of complex urethral reconstruction. In cases in which reconstruction can be accomplished by primary closure, the mucosa and periurethral fascia should be maintained as individual layers. Vaginal epithelium or labial tissue can be

harvested and rotated into place for additional coverage or urethral replacement in cases of stricture. Simultaneous pubovaginal sling placement is advocated in cases of intrinsic sphincter deficiency and incontinence to improve postoperative outcomes after flap urethroplasty for treatment of stricture disease. When distal urethral obstruction is found, the most definitive method of repair is distal urethrectomy and advancement meatoplasty.

REFERENCES

1. Wilson TS, Lemack GE, Zimmern PE. Management of intrinsic sphincteric deficiency in women. J Urol 2003;169:1662–9.
2. Zimmern PE, Hadley HR, Leach GE, et al. Transvaginal closure of the bladder neck and placement of a suprapubic catheter for destroyed urethra after long-term indwelling catheterization. J Urol 1985; 134:554–6.
3. Khoury AE, Agarwal SK, Bagli D, et al. Concomitant modified bladder neck closure and Mitrofanoff urinary diversion. J Urol 1999;162:1746–8.
4. Castera R, Podesta ML, Ruarte A, et al. 10-Year experience with artificial urinary sphincter in children and adolescents. J Urol 2001;165:2373–6.
5. Herndon CDA, Rink RC, Shaw MBK, et al. The Indiana experience with artificial urinary sphincters in children and young adults. J Urol 2003;169: 650–4.
6. Scott FB. The use of the artificial sphincter in the treatment of urinary incontinence in the female patient. Urol Clin North Am 1985;12:305–8.
7. Thomas K, Venn SN, Mundy AR. Outcome of the artificial urinary sphincter in female patients. J Urol 2002;167:1720–2.
8. Long RL, Barrett DM. Artificial sphincter: abdominal approach. In: Female urology. Philadelphia: WB Saunders; 1996. p. 419–27.
9. Wang Y, Hadley HR. Artificial sphincter: transvaginal approach. In: Female urology. Philadelphia: WB Saunders; 1996. p. 428–34.
10. Hartanto VH, Nitti VW. Recent advances in management of female lower urinary tract trauma. Curr Opin Urol 2003;13:279–84.
11. Palou J, Caparros J, Vicente J. Use of proximal-based vaginal flap in stricture of the female urethra. Urol 1996;47:747–9.
12. Flisser AJ, Blaivas JG. Outcome of urethral reconstructive surgery in a series of 74 women. J Urol 2003;169:2246–9.
13. Hemal AK, Dorairajan LN, Gupta NP. Posttraumatic complete and partial loss of urethra with pelvic fracture in girls: an appraisal of management. J Urol 2000;163:282–7.

14. Blaivas JG, Heritz DM. Reconstruction of the damaged urethra. In: Raz S, editor. Female urology. Philadelphia: WB Saunders; 1996 p. 584–97.

15. Bruce RG, El-Galley RES, Galloway NTM. Use of rectus abdominis muscle flap for the treatment of complex and refractory urethrovaginal fistulas. J Urol 2000;163:1212–5.

16. Amundsen CL, Flynn BJ, Webster GD. Urethral erosion after synthetic and nonsynthetic pubovaginal slings: differences in management and continence outcome. J Urol 2003;170:134–7.

Female Urethral Diverticula

Harriette M. Scarpero, MD[a],*, Roger R. Dmochowski, MD[b],
Patrick B. Leu, MD[c]

KEYWORDS

- Urethral diverticulum • Cystourethroscopy
- Voiding cystourethrogram (VCUG)

Surgical excision is the definitive treatment of urethral diverticulum (UD) and the only reasonable surgical option for treating midurethral and proximal UD. Transvaginal excision of a urethral diverticulum previously has been described, and there has been little variance in technique. The description provided in this article does not differ significantly from previous ones, but it offers some practical guidance in adjusting technique to accommodate commonly encountered difficult clinical scenarios.

PREOPERATIVE PLANNING

The diagnosis of a UD is made by history, physical examination, and radiography. Positive pressure urethrography with a double balloon catheter largely has been replaced by alternative imaging methods. A voiding cystourethrogram (VCUG) and transvaginal ultrasound are readily available and commonly used imaging modalities in cases of UD. The diagnosis and surgical management of UD has been enhanced by the application of MRI to the female pelvis (**Fig. 1**). In many centers, MRI has become the imaging study of choice for the evaluation of suspected UD. It is favored because of its multiplanar capabilities and tissue-specific high signal to noise. Other benefits of this study are that the patient does not need to be catheterized and does not need to void for the study. The patient is not exposed to ionizing radiation, and the study can be completed within only three breath-hold sequences.

Although urethral imaging protocols may vary between centers, in most cases the study uses high-resolution, fast spin echo and T_2 weighted sequences. On a T_2 weighted image, the diverticulum appears as a hyperintense, well-circumscribed fluid collection that partially or circumferentially surrounds the urethra. The diverticular wall retains a low-signal intensity, and the neck of the diverticulum is seen as a disruption in the circumferential continuity of the diverticular wall. MRI has a sensitivity of 100% for UD, compared with 69% and 70% for VCUG and urethroscopy, respectively.[1] MRI provides better spatial orientation of the proximity of the diverticulum to the bladder neck and improved ability to assess any anterior extension or circumferentiality of the UD compared with VCUG. For these reasons, MRI may be useful for the planning the surgical treatment of recurrent diverticuli or other complex cases.

Paradoxical incontinence, or the loss of urine from the UD with stress maneuvers, resolves with excision of the UD, but concomitant stress urinary incontinence requires additional treatment. In one study, stress urinary incontinence may have been the initial symptom of UD in as many as 62% of female subjects.[2] Preoperative videourodynamics (VUDS) can be helpful in distinguishing paradoxical incontinence from stress urinary incontinence, because leakage can be visualized across the bladder neck versus from the diverticulum. It may identify any detrusor abnormality that is responsible for current lower urinary tract symptoms and could persist after surgery, such

A version of this article was previously published in the *Atlas of the Urologic Clinics of North America* 12:2.
[a] Associated Urologists, 4230 Harding Road, Suite 521, Nashville, TN 37205, USA
[b] Department of Urologic Surgery, Vanderbilt University Medical Center, Room A 1302, Medical Center North, Nashville, TN 37232, USA
[c] The Urology Center, P.C., 111 South 90th Street, Omaha, NE 68114, USA
* Corresponding author.
E-mail address: hscarpero@comcast.net

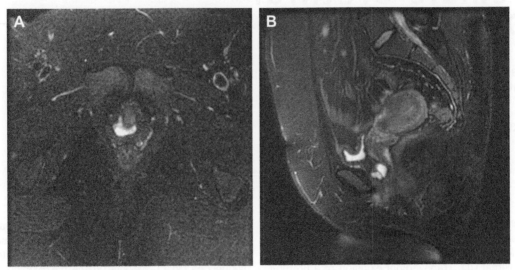

Fig. 1. MRI of complex UD. (*A*) Coronal view of the UD demonstrates that the UD is predominantly posterior but tracks up the right side of the urethra. (*B*) Sagittal view shows the posterior portion of the UD and its large dorsolateral extension.

as involuntary detrusor contractions. The authors typically perform VUDS before surgery in all patients with incontinence.

After the diagnosis is confirmed radiographically, preoperative preparation should include sterilization of the urine and resolution of any acute suppuration and inflammation of the UD with a short course of appropriate antibiotics.

TRANSVAGINAL EXCISION OF URETHRAL DIVERTICULUM
Step One: Cystourethroscopy

Cystourethroscopy may be done in the office before surgery or delayed until the time of surgery. Definitive localization of the diverticular ostium before surgery is helpful, but many women have considerable pain from the UD. In this circumstance, urethroscopy without anesthesia is painful and unlikely to be an optimal opportunity to thoroughly examine the urethral mucosa. A thorough endoscopic evaluation of the urethra should be made using a 0° or 30° lens and a short-beaked cystoscope (Sasche sheath or 17-Fr sheath). If the diverticulum is visible from the vaginal side, it may be compressed to locate the ostium. Expressed contents of the UD into the urethral lumen may identify its site. Ostia typically are found on the floor of the distal two thirds of the urethra between the 4 and 8 o'clock positions. In many instances, however, the ostium cannot be identified easily. The trigone and ureteral orifices are examined. Any distortion of the orifices or intertrigonal ridge could suggest an ectopic ureterocele that should be investigated further

before excision of the vaginal wall mass that previously was suspected to be an UD.

Step Two: Setup, Exposure, and Incision

On leaving the bladder full after cystourethroscopy, a suprapubic catheter may be placed with the aid of a Lowsley retractor (**Fig. 2**). The suprapubic tube can be used to fill the bladder for postoperative VCUG. If there is any evidence of exstravasation, the suprapubic tube can be left in place for

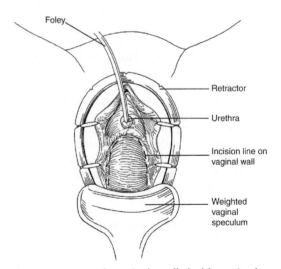

Fig. 2. Setup and vaginal wall incision. A ring retractor is used to retract the labia and vaginal wall as the vaginal incision is made. An inverted U-shaped incision is made from the bladder neck to just proximal to the urethral meatus.

bladder drainage, preventing the need to recatheterize. A 14-Fr Foley catheter is placed in the urethra, and a weighted vaginal speculum is used to retract the posterior vaginal wall.

A Scott ring retractor (Lonestar) provides excellent retraction of the vaginal walls and tissue flaps during UD excision and can be placed before the incision is made. An inverted U-shaped incision is made on the anterior vaginal wall. The apex of the incision is placed just proximal to the meatus. A vaginal wall flap is mobilized off of the periurethral and perivesical fascia to the level of the bladder neck.

Step Three: Development of the Periurethral Flaps

The periurethral fascia is incised transversely with a 15-blade scalpel over the area of the diverticulum (**Fig. 3**). Flaps are raised proximally and distally with Metzanbaum scissors. Care should be taken to preserve this tissue as best as possible so that it may be used as another layer of closure. In cases of recurrent or large diverticula, the periurethral tissue may be tenuous. Once mobilized, the hooks of the Scott retractor can be placed gently on these flaps for better exposure of the UD.

Step Four: Dissection and Excision of the Diverticular Sac

The diverticular sac is grasped gently with delicate forceps and dissected fully to the level of its neck (**Fig. 4**). When the sac is freed on all sides, it is amputated. A urethral defect through which the Foley catheter is visible may be created. A classic recommendation for UD excision has been to avoid entering the sac prematurely because such an action may make dissection more difficult; however, when the neck cannot be delineated fully or the sac is too attenuated to avoid its perforation, it may be necessary to open the sac and urethra longitudinally to search for the ostium. The opened floor of the urethra can be examined closely and probed with a lacrimal duct probe, or its equivalent, until the ostia are identified and the affected portion of urethra is excised.

If the sac is extended anteriorly, this portion must be excised, which requires some mobilization of the urethra on its lateral borders to peel off the sac anteriorly. In cases of large UD, complete excision of the sac requires extensive dissection under the trigone, jeopardizing integrity of the ureters and bladder base. In these situations, it may be prudent to leave the most proximal portion of the sac in place.

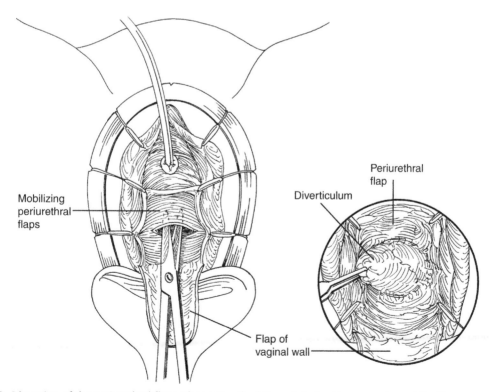

Mobilizing periurethral flaps

Flap of vaginal wall

Diverticulum

Periurethral flap

Fig. 3. Dissection of the periurethral flaps. The periurethral tissue is incised transversely, and the flaps are created proximally and distally.

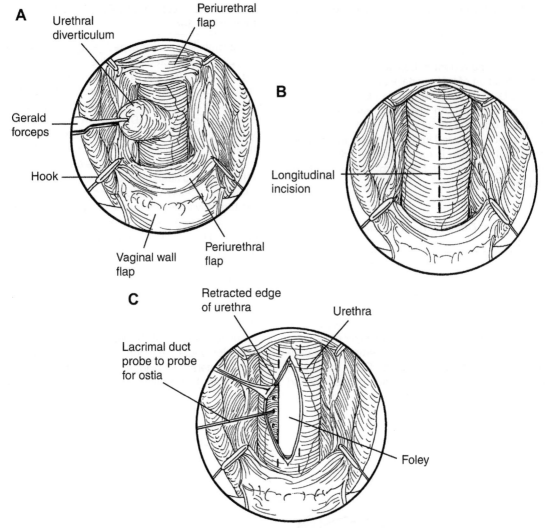

Fig. 4. Excision of the UD. (*A*) After dissecting the periurethral flaps, the UD is identified, dissected down to its neck, and amputated. (*B*) If the UD and ostia cannot be identified, the floor of the urethra can be opened longitudinally. (*C*) The floor of the urethra is probed for ostia, and the affected portion is excised.

Step Five: Closure of the Layers

The key to a successful closure is to ensure a watertight suture line under no tension and with no overlapping of suture lines (**Figs. 5** and **6**). The urethra is closed with a 4-0 running absorbable suture. To ensure watertightness, the clinician can insert an infant feeding tube into the urethra alongside the Foley catheter, inject methylene blue through the tube, and check for any leak of blue fluid from the suture line. The periurethral flaps are closed transversely with a running 3-0 absorbable suture. If these flaps are thin, a Martius flap can be used to cover the urethral closure and provide another layer of vascularized tissue. The vaginal incision is closed with a running 2-0 absorbable suture. Other indications for use of a Martius graft include the following:

> Fibrotic and scarred tissues
> Absence of periurethral fascia
> Recurrent diverticula
> Complicated repair (eg, circumferential diverticulum).

POSTOPERATIVE CARE

After surgery, the patient is maintained on intravenous antibiotics overnight and in the morning is changed to oral antibiotics, which are continued until the urethral catheter is removed. Oral anticholinergics are used liberally to prevent bladder

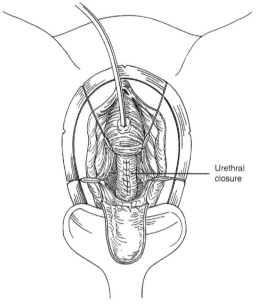

Urethral closure

Fig. 5. Longitudinal closure of the urethra. The urethra is closed with a running 4-0 absorbable suture around a 14-Fr Foley catheter. A smaller catheter may be used if the urethral defect is too large to obtain a tension-free anastomosis around the 14-Fr Foley catheter.

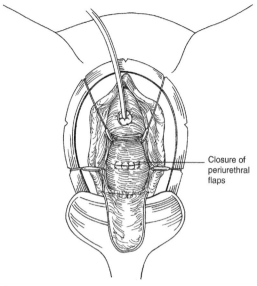

Closure of periurethral flaps

Fig. 6. Transverse closure of the periurethral flaps. The periurethral flaps are closed transversely to avoid overlapping the urethral suture line. If the periurethral flaps are thin, a Martius flap may be brought in for additional coverage.

spasm. In uncomplicated UD excision, a VCUG is performed between postoperative days 7 and 10. It may be delayed for 2 to 3 weeks in cases of complicated repairs. If the vaginal incision is healing well and no exstravasation is seen, the suprapubic tube can be removed when the patient is voiding well and residual volumes are low. If exstravasation is seen, no attempt should be made to recatheterize the urethra, which could disrupt the delicate urethral repair. The suprapubic tube can be kept open for drainage, and a repeat VCUG can be performed in 1 week.

CONCOMITANT PUBOVAGINAL SLING SURGERY

The wisdom of placing an autologous fascial sling at the time of urethral repair has been questioned and substantiated in a few small series.[3,4] The sling is placed over the urethral and periurethral closure and often overlaps these suture lines at least partially. Results indicate that a concomitant pubovaginal sling does not seem to increase the rate of erosion of the sling or infection. The postoperative cure rates in these studies varied from 88% to 100%.[3,4] The safety and efficacy of other sling materials or alternate sling placement is not known and cannot be supported. The use of artificial materials or foreign bodies, such as bone anchors, is discouraged because of the risk for infection.

When a sling is placed in the setting of urethral diverticulectomy, the suspension sutures should be placed before manipulation or decompression of the UD to avoid contamination of the sutures. The vaginal dissection is performed as is done for a standard bladder neck sling. The endopelvic fascia is perforated, and the sutures are carried through the retropubic space with the surgeon's preferred needle passers. Cystoscopy is performed to confirm ureteral patency and lack of perforation of the bladder. By performing these steps before UD excision, additional manipulation of the urethral repair can be avoided. A large UD could be entered during passage of the sutures; it is best to decompress the UD by needle aspiration before dissection to avoid gross spillage of infected contents into the operative field. It is also reasonable to delay treatment of stress incontinence until after repair of the UD.

APPROACH TO THE CIRCUMFERENTIAL DIVERTICULUM

The circumferential UD presents a difficult problem. Total excision leaves an extensive gap that must be reconstructed. Rovner and Wein[5] published their experience with the surgical treatment of circumferential UD. Their technique provides access to the dorsal wall of the urethra and requires a partial urethrectomy in some cases. Urethral continuity is reestablished by diverticular sac urethroplasty or end-to-end urethroplasty. Pain resolved in eight patients (mean follow-up, 19 months). De novo stress urinary incontinence, fistula, and urethral stricture occurred in one case each. One UD recurrence occurred at 37 months.

OUTCOMES AND COMPLICATIONS

Few large series have reported results of UD excision (**Table 1**). Complications of excision include the following:

    Urethral fistula
    Urethral stricture
    UD recurrence
    De novo stress urinary incontinence
    De novo urgency.

Ganabathi and colleagues[2] reviewed 63 women who underwent UD excision over 10 years. Of these women, 56 had a transvaginal diverticulectomy using a three-layer closure. Twenty-seven concomitant bladder neck suspensions were performed. At a mean follow-up of 70 months, 48 women (85.7%) were cured of their presenting complaint. Reported complications included two small recurrent diverticula and one urethrovaginal fistula. The rate of incontinence among women who underwent diverticulectomy alone was 10%, compared with 22% in women who underwent diverticulectomy and bladder neck suspension. Romanzi and colleagues[4] studied 35 women who underwent diverticulectomy with a pubovaginal sling when indicated. Pain was eradicated postoperatively in all but 2 of 22 patients complaining of pain. None of the patients who underwent a concomitant sling procedure had postoperative incontinence, and only one patient developed de novo stress incontinence. In two series examining the outcomes of diverticulectomy with pubovaginal sling, cure rates for stress incontinence ranged from 88% to 100%. No sling erosion was reported, and the residual or recurrent diverticula rates ranged from 12% to 14%. These outcomes

suggest that there is no increased risk for complication with the use of an autologous pubovaginal sling at the time of urethral diverticulectomy.

Excision of UD may be complicated by many of the problems encountered in all types of surgery (eg, bleeding, infection). Significant bleeding is uncommon and can be prevented by careful attention to dissection within the proper planes and use of electrocautery. Placement of a vaginal pack after surgery can be used as a tamponade of vaginal oozing. In some cases, the diverticulum may harbor bacteria or contaminated fluid. Patients should receive a short course of oral antibiotics before surgery. Intravenous antibiotics and copious antibiotic irrigation should be used throughout the procedure. Excision and repair should not be attempted in the suppurative UD. If the infection cannot be cleared by antibiotics alone, it is best to treat the UD with incision and drainage and to perform definitive excision and repair at a later date.

In cases of recurrent, multiple, or large anteriorly reaching diverticula, a sizeable portion of urethra may need to be excised. Closure of the urethra around a 14-Fr catheter may be difficult when the urethral defect is large. In this case, the urethra may be mobilized to expose more of the urethral wall, and closure can be completed over an 8-Fr feeding tube. Urethral stricture is a known complication of UD excision and is a risk when closure is performed over a smaller feeding tube. In these more complex cases, particularly in patients who underwent previous operations, the periurethral tissues may be of poor quality. A Martius flap provides a healthy graft for interposition between the urethral and vaginal incisions in such cases.

The most dreaded complication of UD excision is urethrovaginal fistula. Its reported incidence ranges from 0.9% to 8%.[2] Repair of a fistula is undertaken after the inflammation has subsided; generally, this change requires 2 to 3 months. A Martius flap often is used as an extra layer of vascularized tissue to improve the chance of successful healing.

Table 1
Comparison of series results of transvaginal excision of UD

Author	Mean FU (mo)	No. of patients	Postoperative SUI	Postoperative fistula	Recurrence
Ganabathi	70	56	9	1	2
Romanzi	39	35	1	NA	NA
Swierzewski	17	14	0	0	1
Faerber	23	16	2	0	2

Abbreviation: NA, information not specifically addressed in results.

Diverticula may recur in situations of continued infection, excessive tension on the repair, or failure to remove all of the diverticular sac and its neck. The best preventive approaches are preoperative preparation with control of infection before surgery, detailed diagnostic imaging to determine the number and extent of diverticula, and meticulous surgical technique.

The reported incidence of stress urinary incontinence after diverticulectomy ranges from 4% to 20%. The mechanism is believed to be dissection of the urethral support mechanisms or damage to the urinary sphincter during excision of the UD. Any complaint of urinary incontinence after excision of UD should be evaluated to rule out a urethrovaginal or vesicovaginal fistula.

SUMMARY

Transvaginal excision of UD is the gold-standard therapy, but success depends on proper staging by determination of the extent and number of diverticula and attention to surgical technique. MRI provides excellent visualization of the UD in several planes and has greatly improved the ability to assess this condition. No debate exists regarding proper surgical technique. The principles of complete excision of the UD, watertight and tension-free closure, and no overlapping suture lines are endorsed by all surgical descriptions. It has been shown that the concomitant performance of pubovaginal sling surgery does not increase the risks for erosion into the urethra and fistula formation.

REFERENCES

1. Kim B, Hricak H, Tanagho E. Diagnosis of urethral diverticula in women: value of MG imaging. AJR Am J Roentgenol 1993;161:809–15.
2. Ganabathi K, Leach GE, Zimmern PE, et al. Experience with the management of urethral diverticulum in 63 women. J Urol 1994;152:1445–52.
3. Faerber GJ. Urethral diverticulectomy and pubovaginal sling for simultaneous treatment of urethral diverticulum and intrinsic sphincter deficiency. Tech Urol 1998;4:192–7.
4. Romanzi LJ, Groutz A, Blaivas JG. Urethral diverticulum in women: diverse presentations resulting in diagnostic delay and mismanagement. J Urol 2000; 164:428–33.
5. Rovner ES, Wein AJ. Diagnosis and reconstruction of the dorsal or circumferential urethral diverticulum. J Urol 2003;170:82–6.

FURTHER READINGS

Blander DS, Rovner ES, Schnall MD, et al. Endoluminal magnetic resonance imaging in the evaluation of urethral diverticula in women. Urology 2001;57: 660–5.

Neitlich JD, Foster HE, Glickman MG, et al. Detection of urethral diverticula in women: comparison of a high resolution fast spin echo technique with double balloon urethrography. J Urol 1998;159:408–10.

Swierzewski JJ, McGuire EJ. Pubovaginal sling for treatment of female stress urinary incontinence complicated by urethral diverticulum. J Urol 1993;149: 1012–4.

Male Slings in the Treatment of Sphincteric Incompetence

J. Christian Winters, MD

KEYWORDS

- Prostatectomy • Bulbourethral sling
- Bone-anchored perineal sling
- Prostatic urethral sling • Neurogenic bladder

The incidence of urinary incontinence is approximately 1% to 3% after prostatectomy for benign disease,[1] and after radical prostatectomy, the incidence has been reported to range from 2.5% to 87%.[2,3] This wide discrepancy is a result of varying definitions of incontinence and inconsistent methods of data acquisition. The timing of studies is important, as urinary control may improve with time. Most patients have some degree of incontinence immediately after catheter removal, but a progressive reduction in incontinence may occur up to 1 year after prostatectomy. There is little dispute that the occurrence of incontinence after prostatectomy has a significant negative impact on a patient's quality of life. In a questionnaire-based study, Herr[4] discovered that incontinence adversely affected the quality of life in 26% of patients, and in a separate survey, patients who underwent radical prostatectomy scored significantly worse on a scale evaluating urinary function compared with controls. Patients should be screened after prostatectomy for these symptoms, which are likely to have a detrimental effect on quality of life.

CAUSE OF INCONTINENCE AFTER PROSTATECTOMY

Urinary leakage may occur as a result of an abnormality of bladder or sphincteric function. Bladder dysfunction has been documented as the predominant cause of incontinence after prostatectomy.[5]

Subsequent reports have disputed this finding, noting that isolated sphincter dysfunction is the major cause of incontinence after prostate surgery.[6–8] On closer review, many studies documenting a high incidence of bladder dysfunction as the sole cause of incontinence contain a large percentage of patients who have undergone transurethral resection of the prostate (TURP). Bladder dysfunction frequently exists before surgery and may persist after surgery. After undergoing radical prostatectomy, the predominant cause of incontinence is an isolated intrinsic sphincter deficiency. Bladder dysfunction may occur after radical prostatectomy but usually occurs with concomitant sphincter dysfunction. Mixed incontinence, the combination of sphincteric incompetence and bladder dysfunction, that occurs after radical prostatectomy has a reported incidence of approximately 20% to 40%.[5–7] Bladder dysfunction may improve over time. In patients undergoing urodynamics at least 1 year after radical prostatectomy, sphincteric dysfunction is the most likely cause.[6] Approximately one third of these patients may have coexisting bladder dysfunction, which could greatly affect treatment outcomes. After TURP, a higher incidence of bladder dysfunction is likely present, particularly if studied sooner than 1 year after surgery. As most clinicians have experienced, symptoms do not accurately predict diagnosis. Urodynamic studies are important to characterize the lower urinary tract dysfunction that is present.[7]

A version of this article was previously published in the *Atlas of the Urologic Clinics of North America* 12:2.
Department of Urology, Ochsner Clinic Foundation, AT-4, 1514 Jefferson Highway, New Orleans, LA 70121, USA
E-mail address: cwinters@ochsner.org

Urol Clin N Am 38 (2011) 73–81
doi:10.1016/j.ucl.2010.12.010

EVALUATION OF POSTPROSTATECTOMY INCONTINENCE

A focused history should include detailed information about the precipitants of urinary leakage. One should note when the onset of leakage occurred after surgery and whether incontinence was present before surgery. Associated voiding symptoms are important factors. Validated incontinence questionnaires are an easy way to objectively quantify the severity of incontinence symptoms. Daytime and nighttime pad use should be documented, and a pad weight test should be considered to more accurately quantify urinary leakage. Treatment options may be chosen on the basis of incontinence severity, and these tools are helpful in determining incontinence severity. A physical examination should include rectal examination to assess the size and consistency of the prostate. Sphincter tone should be assessed, and the quality of sphincter contraction should be analyzed by having the patient compress the sphincter. The patient should have an adequate localized contraction of the sphincter muscles without excessive use of accessory muscles. One should observe for the presence of leakage. Does the patient passively leak with standing or when prompted to cough? A urinalysis and residual urine should be obtained, and prostate-specific antigen testing should be considered.

Cystourethroscopy should be performed to rule out the presence of urethral stricture disease or bladder neck contracture. Inspection of the sphincter may reveal gross abnormalities, but cystoscopic examination does not determine sphincter function. After TURP, absence of the verumontanum suggests sphincteric injury, which should prompt further study. After radical prostatectomy, an urethrovesical anastomosis that is at the level of the external sphincter may suggest impairment of the sphincter mechanism.

Urodynamic evaluation is essential to determine the cause of incontinence after prostatectomy and must be performed in patients for whom invasive therapy is considered. The investigation should provide information regarding bladder and sphincteric function during filling and should assess bladder contractility and flow during voiding. A multichannel urodynamic study most optimally provides this information. The use of electromyography of the pelvic floor is indicated in cases complicated by neurologic dysfunction. Urethral pressure profilometry can provide information regarding urethral closing pressures and functional urethral length. Videourodynamics provides the most complete evaluation, combining the anatomic detail of voiding cystourethrography with the functional assessment of pressure-flow studies.

During bladder filling, information regarding detrusor overactivity, compliance abnormalities, sensation, and cystometric capacity specifically is noted. The Valsalva leak point pressure (VLPP) is determined. If leakage occurs during straining in the absence of an increase in detrusor pressure, sphincteric incompetence is demonstrated. The exact numerical value of the VLPP has not been correlated to the severity of incontinence but is an area of considerable research. As new treatment options for sphincteric incompetence in men emerge, VLPP values may facilitate proper selection of patients for different procedures. The filling phase of the urodynamic study is critical, as one should determine whether the bladder is stable with normal storage pressures and of adequate storage capacity. Patients with an abnormality of compliance, significant motor detrusor overactivity, or decreased cystometric capacity should be offered initial therapy that is directed at bladder management. If bladder storage abnormalities remain undetected, treatment for sphincteric incompetence may fail and/or detrimental changes to the upper urinary tract may develop. The voiding phase of the pressure-flow study provides valuable information regarding bladder contractility and voiding dynamics.

TREATMENT OF SPHINCTERIC INCOMPETENCE WITH THE BULBOURETHRAL SLING

The many options in the management of patients with incontinence after prostatectomy include: pharmacotherapy, pelvic floor physiotherapy, electrical stimulation, and urethral injection therapy. The gold standard of the surgical management of postprostatectomy incontinence is the artificial urinary sphincter. Patient satisfaction rates are high after artificial sphincter implantation; however, problems such as urethral erosion and tissue atrophy, which require reoperation, may occur. Although modifications to the cuff design may reduce the overall incidence of revisions, some patients will continue to require reoperation, especially if the sphincter has been implanted for a long time. For these reasons, the concept of sling procedures to provide urethral compression has emerged. Although sling procedures in women and men differ, they involve the same principles to create broad-based uniaxial compressive forces on the urethra to maintain continence.

Schaeffer and colleagues[9] described a male bulbourethral sling procedure using synthetic bolsters passed beneath the bulbar urethra and suspended by the rectus fascia. A midline perineal incision is created, and three tetra-fluoroethylene bolsters are placed below the bulbar urethra. A small suprapubic incision is created, and a modified Stamey needle is passed from the suprapubic incision into the perineal incision. Nonabsorbable sutures that are attached to the bolsters are transferred to the suprapubic incision and tied over the rectus fascia.[10] Bone anchors that are inserted into the pubic bone can be added for additional support. Intraoperative measurements of urethral pressures or abdominal leak point pressures can be performed to assist in judging appropriate sling tension. This procedure demonstrated that bulbourethral slings can be used successfully to treat postprostatectomy incontinence.

Technique of the Bone-Anchored Perineal Sling Procedure

Many surgeons perform a bone-anchored sling implanted by way of a perineal incision. Advantages of this approach include a single incision, stable anchor fixation to the bony pelvis, and no risk for bladder injury.[11,12] The basic principles of this procedure are stable fixation of the sling material to the bony pelvis, broad-based compression of the urethra, and preservation of the bulbospongiosus muscle.[13] If these principles are met, compression of the urethra facilitating continence should be created with little risk for erosion or urinary retention.

The patient is positioned in the dorsal lithotomy position and, a Foley catheter is inserted. The operation is begun by creating a midline perineal incision (**Fig. 1**). The bulbospongiosus muscle is identified and preserved. The dissection proceeds laterally

toward the medial aspect of the descending pubic ramus, which is located by palpation (**Fig. 2**). The junction of the descending pubic ramus and the pubic tubercle should be located. During this dissection, a finder needle can assist in localizing the bone (**Fig. 3**) under the soft tissues. The first set of bone anchors should be placed as high on the pubic ramus (at the level of the pubic symphysis) as possible. Electrocautery and scissor dissection should continue until the soft tissues are cleared from the periosteum, allowing direct visualization and precise anchor placement into the bone. Two or three sets of anchors are to be implanted into the bone. I prefer positioning three anchors on each side, as this method facilitates stronger fixation and allows for more compression. Several investigators successfully used two anchors on each side. Anchor positioning starts at the level of the pubic symphysis and proceeds caudally toward the ischial spines (**Fig. 4**). The anchors are positioned just over 1 cm apart, proceeding caudally. Anchors are implanted in a similar location on the contralateral side. The anchors are placed using a straight drill, placing anchors preloaded with polypropylene sutures. The sling graft is fashioned in a trapezoid shape to accommodate the shape of the bony pelvis. The graft should measure approximately $4 \times 6 \times 4$ cm. Various graft materials have been used, including cadaveric fascia, cadaveric dermis, polypropylene mesh, and silicone. I prefer a synthetic graft, as biologic materials may tear or stretch excessively when achieving the proper compression. The graft material is attached to the three anchors on one side. The material then is positioned on the opposite side after determining proper tension. Securing a clamp to the graft allows proper positioning of the graft on the bone (**Fig. 5**). The Foley catheter is withdrawn into the fossa navicularis where the balloon is reinflated. A retrograde perusion test is performed by connecting an infusion bag of normal saline, and the drip chamber is positioned 60 cm above the pubic symphysis (see **Fig. 5**). The sling is positioned on the contralateral bone with enough tension to stop the infusion of saline. At this point, the sutures are brought out through the graft medial to the clamp (**Fig. 6**). A single throw of the prolene suture is placed over a silk suture. This step allows reversal of the knot if the suture needs to be repositioned. The retrograde perfusion pressure is repeated to insure a retrograde perfusion pressure of at least 60 cm of water. The sutures are tied, and any excess graft is trimmed (**Fig. 7**). The wound is closed in multiple layers after copious irrigation with antibiotic solution. The catheter may be removed the next day, and intermittent catheterization may be performed if the patient is unable to void.

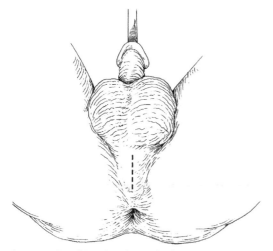

Fig. 1. Perineal incision for male sling.

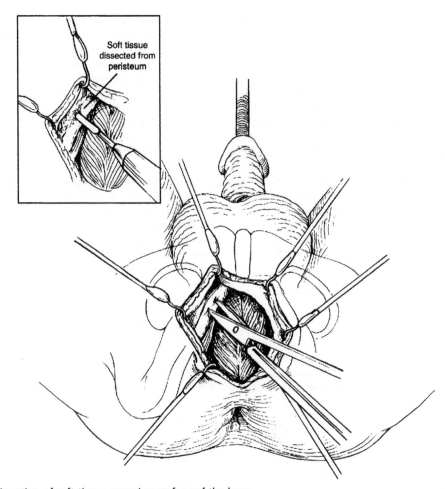

Soft tissue
dissected from
peristeum

Fig. 2. Dissection of soft tissue, exposing surface of the bone.

Several investigators have noted dry and improved rates of 76% to 86% after undergoing the bone-anchored bulbourethral sling procedure. Follow-up in studies has been short term, ranging from a mean follow-up of 6 months to 12.2 months.[13,14] Few complications have been noted. Urinary retention was observed in 0% to 33.3% of patients and resolved within 7 days in all patients. Transient scrotal numbness has been reported in a small number of patients and resolved in 6 weeks. One scrotal hematoma has been reported. No osseous complications (osteomyelitis or osteitis pubis) have been reported, and no cases of urethral erosion have been identified.[15] Urinary urgency and urge incontinence were identified in a small number of patients who responded well to anticho-linergic medication. No sexual dysfunction has been reported. Artificial sphincter placement after sling failure has been performed without difficulty.

A sling does not preclude subsequent sphincter placement.

TREATMENT OF NEUROGENIC BLADDER WITH THE PROSTATIC URETHRAL SLING

In patients with neurogenic bladder dysfunction, impaired urethral resistance may occur, particu-larly in patients with lesions that disrupt the thora-columbar outflow. Many of these patients have a wide open bladder neck and proximal urethral sphincter. Urodynamics confirm low VLPP. These patients may require more outlet resistance than bulbourethral slings may generate. The mainstay of therapy has been the artificial urinary sphincter or bladder neck reconstruction. The rates of infec-tion and erosion of the artificial urinary sphincter are higher in patients with a neurogenic bladder than those with postprostatectomy incontinence,

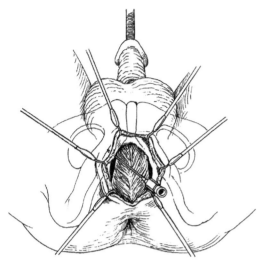

Fig. 3. Finder needle to assist in localization of the bone.

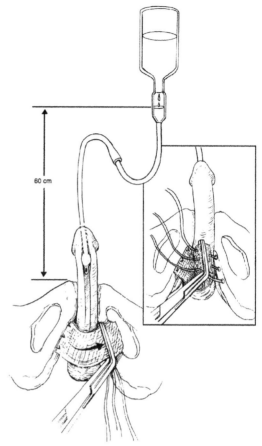

and patients with neurogenic lower urinary tract dysfunction tend to be younger, increasing the likelihood of artificial sphincter revision. A fascial bladder neck sling may provide an alternative approach and can be performed safely at the time of a bladder augmentation procedure.[16]

Evaluation of Patients with Neurogenic Bladder

As in patients with postprostatectomy incontinence, the evaluation in patients with neurogenic

Fig. 5. Adjustment of sling tension. After fixation of sling on one side, a right-angle clamp is used to place the sling on the pubic bone. With appropriate tension, the infusion of saline into the urethra should be prevented on retrograde perfusion that is set at 60 cm of water. The opposite sling sutures are placed medial to the clamp, insuring that proper tension is placed. The perfusion test may be repeated before replacing the Foley catheter in the bladder.

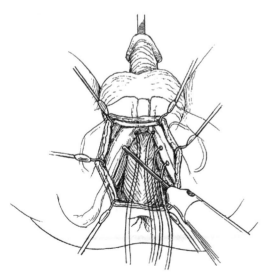

Fig. 4. Anchor placement into the medial aspect of the descending pubic rami. Location of distal anchors at the level of the symphysis is shown.

bladder should stress symptom assessment and diagnostic testing to determine bladder and sphincteric function. Upper tract evaluation is mandatory. Levels of serum creatinine and electrolytes are determined, and isotope renography is obtained as indicated. Cystoscopy is performed, particularly in patients who are on intermittent catheterization, to rule out urethral stricture, false passages, and bladder pathology. Videourodynamic studies are obtained. It is vital to determine detrusor compliance and detect signs of neurogenic detrusor overactivity. If a compliance persists despite maximal medical therapy, bladder augmentation should be considered at the time of the bladder neck sling

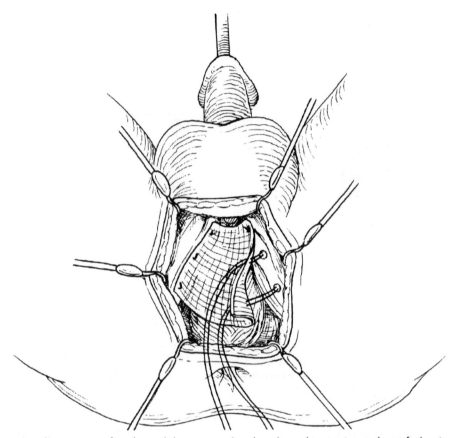

Fig. 6. Securing sling sutures after determining appropriate location using a retrograde perfusion test.

procedure. Sphincteric dysfunction is assessed by measurement of VLPP, which must be obtained in the absence of a detrusor contraction under normal detrusor storage pressures. Fluoroscopy allows for additional anatomic information. The bladder neck should be visualized, and many patients have an open bladder neck at rest in association with low VLPP. The presence of vesicoureteral reflux, which may need correction, should be determined, as should detrusor contractility. Patients with impaired contractility may not be able to empty after bladder neck sling and may need to be prepared for subsequent intermittent catheterization. An artificial sphincter should be considered in these patients, as less resistance is created by the sphincter cuff when opened, facilitating the ability to empty without the need for catheterization.

Technique of the Prostatic Urethral Sling Procedure

Patients undergo a mechanical bowel preparation and are administered broad-spectrum antibiotics before surgery. Patients are positioned supine or in the low lithotomy position. A Foley catheter is inserted in the bladder. I routinely place a rectal catheter to assist in sling placement. The operation may be performed using a midline abdominal incision or a Pfannensteil approach. The space of

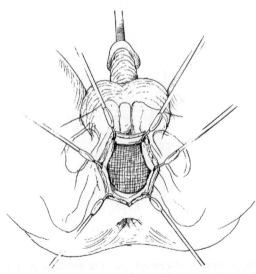

Fig. 7. Graft in position after being secured to both sides of descending pubic rami.

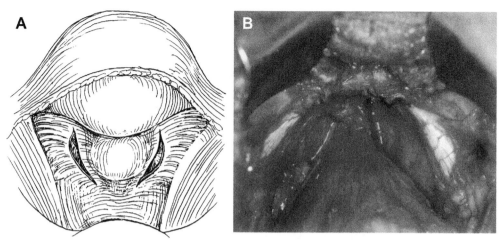

Fig. 8. (*A*) Incision of endopelvic fascia to expose apex of prostate and facilitate dissection of space between rectum and urethra. (*B*) Intraoperative view. Endopelvic fascia is incised on patient's right, facilitating access to apex.

Retzius is developed, and the peritoneum is mobilized cephalad by blunt dissection. The endopelvic fascia is visualized and incised widely (**Fig. 8**). After incision of the endopelvic fascia, the plane between the urethra and rectum is developed. After incision of the endopelvic fascia, this plane often is easily developed bluntly. The previously placed rectal catheter aids in identification of the rectum to avoid injury. If this plane remains difficult to develop, the bladder is opened, and a finger is placed in the urethra to facilitate dissection. A right-angled clamp is placed beneath the urethra, and a penrose drain is positioned into the space for sling placement (**Fig. 9**). Inspection is performed to rule out urethral or rectal injury. Flexible cystoscopy or dilute iodine injection into the rectal catheter may be performed if one is suspicious of injury. Direct inspection should suffice in routine cases. If bladder augmentation is to be performed, it usually is done at this point. An autologous sling, which is harvested through the incision site, generally is chosen. The sling measures 1.5 cm wide and 10 to 12 cm long. It is passed into the space previously created between the urethra and rectum and is crossed at the midline anterior to the urethra and secured to the opposite Cooper's ligament (on one side) with permanent suture. Once this step is completed, the bladder is filled with 250 to 300 mL of normal saline, and the urethral catheter is removed. Manual pressure is placed on the bladder, and the sling is fixed to the contralateral Cooper's ligament in a location that prevents leakage with bladder compression (**Fig. 10**). Patients are catheterized on the table to insure that there will be no difficulty with subsequent

catheterization. The wound is irrigated copiously, and the incision closed.

Success rates of 66% to 83% have been reported in small numbers of patients with a follow-up of approximately 14 months.[17,18] Several reports in pediatric patients also report encouraging success rates and significant increases in leak point pressures after the prostatic urethral sling procedure.[19] Reported complications are rare, and long-term follow-up is needed to determine if this procedure remains a viable alternative to use of an artificial urinary sphincter or bladder neck reconstruction.

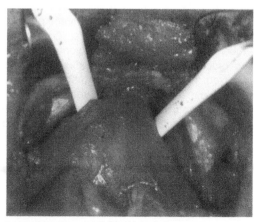

Fig. 9. Penrose drain in space between rectum and urethra. Cooper's ligament is exposed bilaterally.

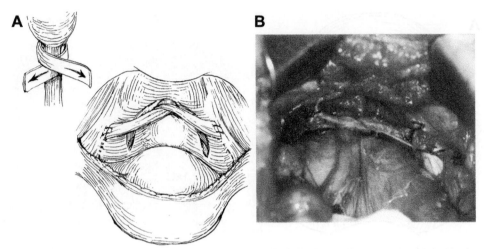

Fig. 10. (*A–B*) Final result. The sling is crossed over at midline and secured to contralateral Cooper's ligament.

SUMMARY

Advances in surgical management of incontinence have led to new alternatives in the management of postprostatectomy incontinence and neurogenic bladder in men. The bone-anchored bulbourethral sling is being used with increasing frequency because of its single-incision approach, prompt return to voiding, and immediate continence. No cases of urethral erosion or tissue atrophy have been reported, and such cases may be unlikely as a result of bulbospongiosus muscle preservation and uniaxial compression of the urethra. Several questions must be answered with future study. It generally is accepted that patients with mild-to-moderate incontinence are appropriate candidates for a male sling, and patients with more severe degrees of incontinence should be treated with an artificial sphincter. Future studies are needed to determine a more objective way to select patients for the most appropriate procedure. Pad testing or leak point pressures perhaps may be used to select patients. Only small numbers of patients have undergone the male sling procedure after radiation, and the results are mixed. It is not yet proven that male slings are durable in patients after undergoing radiation. The most important question remains: Will the high degree of patient satisfaction be maintained in long-term study? Until this question is answered, the artificial urinary sphincter remains the gold-standard treatment of postprostatectomy incontinence. Similar concerns exist regarding the prostatic urethral sling in males with neurogenic bladder dysfunction. A procedure that can achieve long-term correction of intrinsic sphincter deficiency and avoid the potential complications of an artificial sphincter would be a significant advance. Stable fixation of autologous fascia to Cooper's ligament may achieve this result.

Sling procedures in men can be performed with little morbidity and few complications. Early results are encouraging, and high levels of patient satisfaction have been achieved. Men with mild-to-moderate intrinsic sphincteric dysfunction after prostatectomy seem to be appropriate candidates for the bone-anchored bulbourethral sling, and the prostatic urethral sling may be an acceptable substitute in patients with neurogenic bladder with intrinsic sphincteric dysfunction.

REFERENCES

1. Marks J, Light JK. Management of urinary incontinence after prostatectomy. J Urol 1989;142:302–4.
2. Walsh P, Jewett A. Radical surgery for prostate cancer. Cancer 1980;45(7 suppl):1906–11.
3. Rudy D, Woodside J, Crawford E. Urodynamic evaluation of incontinence in patients undergoing modified Campbell radical retropubic prostatectomy: a prospective study. J Urol 1984;132:708–12.
4. Herr H. Quality of life of incontinent men after radical prostatectomy. J Urol 1994;151:652–4.
5. Khan Z, Mieza M, Starer P, et al. Post-prostatectomy incontinence: a urodynamic and fluoroscopic point of view. Urology 1991;38:483–8.
6. Winters J, Appell R, Rackley R. Urodynamic findings in postprostatectomy incontinence. Neurourol Urodynam 1998;17:493–8.
7. Groutz A, Blaivas J, Chaikin D, et al. The pathophysiology of post-radical prostatectomy incontinence: a clinical and videourodynamics study. J Urol 2000;163:1767–70.

8. Scarpero H, Winters J. Postprostatectomy incontinence. In: Appell R, editor. Current clinical urology, voiding dysfunction: diagnosis and treatment. Totowa (NJ): Humana Press; 2001. p. 251–62.

9. Schaeffer A, Clemens J, Ferrari M, et al. The male bulbourethral sling procedure for post-radical prostatectomy incontinence. J Urology 1988;159:1510–5.

10. Kapoor R, Dubey D, Kumar A, et al. Modified bulbar urethral sling procedure for the treatment of male sphincter incontinence. J Endourol 2001;15:545–9.

11. Madjar S, Jacoby K, Giberti C, et al. Bone anchored sling for the treatment of post-prostatectomy incontinence. J Urol 2001;165:72–6.

12. Cespedes R, Jacoby K. Male slings for postprostatectomy incontinence. Tech Urol 2001;7:176–83.

13. Franco N, Baum N. Suburethral sling for male urinary incontinence. Infect Urol 2001;14:10–8.

14. Comiter C. The male sling for stress urinary incontinence: a prospective study. J Urol 2002;167:597–601.

15. Petrou S. Treatment of postprostatectomy incontinence: is the bulbourethral sphincter a viable alternative to the artificial urinary sphincter? Curr Urol Rep 2002;3:360–4.

16. Raz S, McGuire E, Erlich R, et al. Fascial sling to correct male neurogenic sphincter incompetence: the McGuire/Raz approach. J Urol 1995;139:528–31.

17. Daneshmand S, Ginsberg D, Bennet J, et al. Puboprostatic sling repair for treatment of urethral incompetence in adult neurogenic incontinence. J Urol 2003;169:199–202.

18. Kakizaki H, Shibata T, Shinno Y, et al. Fascial sling for the management of urinary incontinence due to sphincter incompetence. J Urol 1995;153:644–7.

19. Nguyen H, Bauer S, Diamond D, et al. Rectus fascia sling for the treatment of neurogenic sphincteric incontinence in boys: Is it safe and effective? J Urol 2001;166:658–61.

Artificial Urinary Sphincter: Lessons Learned

Andrew C. Peterson, MD[a],*, George D. Webster, MB, FRCS[b]

KEYWORDS

- Incontinence • Urodynamic study • Urethroscopy

Since its introduction in 1973 (American Medical Systems [AMS] model 721), the artificial urinary sphincter (AUS) has become a widely accepted therapy, particularly for male urinary incontinence. Over the years, improvements in product design, surgical techniques, and patient selection have led to increased reliability with durable success. The current American Medical Systems model 800 (AMS 800) AUS was introduced in 1983 and has a 20-year history of use. This device has become the gold-standard treatment for incontinence of many causes, including prostatectomy, radiation therapy, neuropathy, and as a part of reconstructive procedures. Outcomes with the device are excellent, and most patients are pleased with the results, an outcome that persists in the long term.[1–3] The authors review their experience with more than 600 AUS devices and discuss practical points concerning surgery and revisions. They describe their routine surgical approach as a means of reporting on technical lessons learned.

PREOPERATIVE EVALUATION

Evaluation of patients for treatment with an AUS starts with a comprehensive office visit, including taking a history and performing a physical examination, urinalysis, and urine culture. Each patient completes a 72-hour voiding diary and a 24-hour urinary pad weight test that is brought to the office visit. The pad-weight study is an invaluable objective measure of the magnitude of the incontinence.

During the office visit, videourodynamics are performed. This step, along with the voiding diary and patient history, helps confirm the factors contributing to the incontinence and identifies factors that may mitigate against a good outcome. Some investigators have suggested that urodynamic study is superfluous to the selection of the patient for implantation, but the authors disagree. Cystoscopy is performed in all patients to evaluate the urethra for a healthy placement site and to exclude urethral strictures and anastomotic contracture.

PREPARATION

The authors attempt to ensure that the urine is sterile and that infected foci are not present the week before surgery. Preoperative antibiotics (an aminoglycoside and cephazolin or vancomycin) are given intravenously. Surgery is conducted under general or spinal anesthesia with the patient in the low lithotomy position and with the entire operative site shaved. Before draping, a 10-minute, iodine-based skin preparation is performed that includes the lower abdomen, genitals, and perineum. A 16-French Foley catheter is placed to drain the bladder and to facilitate identification and dissection of the urethra, which is the first step of the procedure.

CUFF PLACEMENT

The ideal site for placement of the AUS cuff is at the bulbar urethra just proximal to the bifurcation

A version of this article was previously published in the *Atlas of the Urologic Clinics of North America* 12:2.
[a] Division of Urology, Duke University Medical Center, DUMC 3146, Room 1113, Green Zone, Davison Building, Durham, NC 27710, USA
[b] Department of Urologic Surgery, Duke University Medical Center, Box 3146, Durham, NC 27710, USA
* Corresponding author. Medical Corps, Department of the Army, Urology Service, Tacoma, WA 98431–1100.
E-mail address: drew.peterson@duke.edu

Urol Clin N Am 38 (2011) 83–88
doi:10.1016/j.ucl.2010.12.011

of the corporal bodies (**Fig. 1**). Bucks fascia is incised, as it reflects off the bulbar urethra onto the diverging corporal bodies. A tunnel can be made using scissor dissection, dorsal to Buck's fascia over the roof of the urethra as it passes between the separating corporal bodies. A right-angle clamp may be passed atraumatically through this tunnel while avoiding the dorsal aspect of the urethra (**Fig. 2**). Blunt or spread dissection can be hazardous in this area, as it risks the thinning of the urethra or splitting into the urethra. Being posterior to the bifurcation of the corporal bodies is important in that it allows for a safer dissection dorsal to the urethra and presents a larger urethra.

Generally, a 4.0- or 4.5-cm AUS cuff is selected, and a cuff that has the snuggest fit, but is not obstructive, results in better continence (**Fig. 3**). The circumference of the urethra at the dissected site is measured in centimeters to guide selection of cuff size. The authors believe that the measurement should be taken on a bare corpus spongiosum, as intervening fat or muscle rapidly atrophies, causing leakage of the device. Other than when implanting a transcorporal cuff, the cuff size is always smaller than the measured circumference of the urethra, because much of what is measured around the urethra is compressible spongy tissue and because postoperative subcuff atrophy will occur. Although no accurate guide can be given, generally

if the corpus spongiosum measures 5 cm, the authors implant a 4-cm cuff.

The best test of cuff fit is the visual and endoscopic appearance after it has been placed around the urethra. If the measurement was incorrect, it is often obvious (the cuff looks obviously too loose or is strangling the urethra). At this point, the cuff should be changed, regardless of waste of equipment. If the margin of tightness is small, cuff size can be increased by a few millimeters by excising up to 2 mm from inside the tab. Caution must be used in performing this unapproved maneuver, as removing too much from the cuff tab may create a hole that is large enough to cause herniation of the cuff through the tab hole and malfunction of the device. The authors routinely perform urethroscopy after urethral dissection and cuff placement to ensure an absence of dissection injury to the urethra and to confirm good cuff sizing.

The tubing to the AUS cuff is passed from the perineal dissection using a transfer trocar or a tonsil clamp (underneath Colles' fascia and staying close to the pubic bone) to the right lower quadrant abdominal wound where the incision is located for placement of the reservoir and scrotal pump. Throughout the procedure, the operative site and the components periodically and liberally are irrigated with an antibiotic solution.

PRESSURE-REGULATING BALLOON PLACEMENT

A horizontal 5-cm right lower quadrant incision is made in Langer's lines of the abdomen, and the subcutaneous tissue is incised with electrocautery down to the abdominal wall fascia above the inguinal canal. The fascia is incised in the line of its fibers, and the underlying muscle is split to access the preperitoneal space. Limited digital dissection of this space is performed, as the space required for the reservoir is small. The inferior epigastric vessels can be injured during this dissection. A 61- to 70-cm H_2O pressure-regulating balloon is placed into the space and filled with approximately 23 mL of contrast material as recommended by the manufacturer. The authors rarely use the 51- to 60-cm H_2O pressure-regulating balloons or the 71- to 80-cm H_2O pressure-regulating balloons. The abdominal wall fascia is closed around the exiting tube with #1 polyglycolic acid suture.

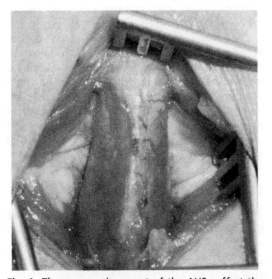

Fig. 1. The proper placement of the AUS cuff at the proximal urethra. The divergent corporal bodies protect the cuff from inadvertent activation when sitting. This location is reached easily with the patient in low lithotomy and can be felt before incision as the area where the urethral catheter is no longer palpable in the perineum.

PUMP PLACEMENT

According to the authors, the most successful technique for accurately locating the pump assembly in the anterior scrotum is, from the inguinal incision, to dissect inferiorly on the level above the abdominal

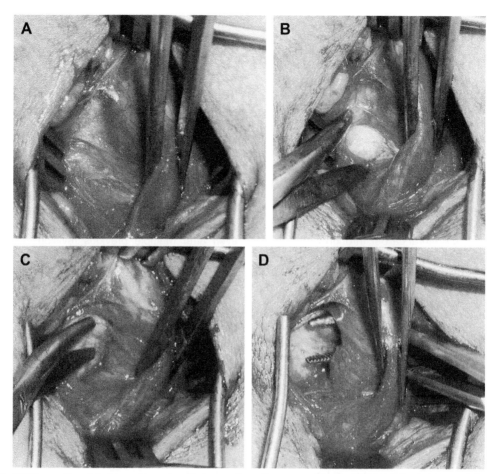

Fig. 2. (*A*) The urethra is held gently and pulled away from the corporal body. (*B*) Buck's fascia is incised sharply as it reflects off of the bulbar urethra. This step allows clean, sharp dissection of the ventral urethra under direct vision (*C*) and provides protection from injury during manipulation (*D*).

wall fascia but deep to Scarpas fascia toward the neck of the scrotum. At the scrotal neck, the fascia is broken through, with the finger tip accessing the anterior scrotum deep to dartos fascia. A finger

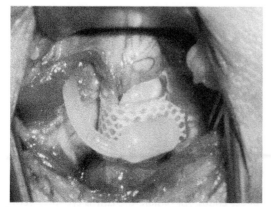

Fig. 3. For good function, the cuff should fit snugly around the bulbar urethra.

placed outside the dependent portion of the scrotum invaginates this skin upward into the inguinal incision, allowing the fascial layers to be stripped off the dartos layer and creating a small pocket for the pump. The pump is placed into that position and held with a Babcock clamp. Pump placement that is too deep may leave the pump adherent to the testicle and difficult to activate. Postoperatively, the pump must be kept low in the scrotum by teaching the patient to pull it down daily and to avoid surgical dressings, underwear, or incontinence products that may dislodge it cephalad. Although the tubings are kink proof, a high pump that is turned on itself is difficult to use.

MAKING THE CONNECTIONS

Connections are performed in the abdominal wound using the quick connectors supplied by the manufacturer. A straight connector attaches the tubing from the pump to the pressure-regulating balloon, and a right-angle connector is used to attach the tubing from the pump to the cuff. Correct tubing length is paramount to maintaining the pump in its dependent scrotal location. If only a single component is replaced after device malfunction, quick connectors should not be used, as they insecurely connect old tubings to new tubings.

All rubber-shodded clamps are removed from the tubing, and the device is tested. Urethroscopy is performed to the level of the cuff. With the cuff closed, a slight blanching of the urethral tissue should indicate adequate coaptation of the device for continence. Under direct endoscopic vision, the cuff is cycled to verify an adequate urethral caliber through which voiding is allowed (**Fig. 4**).

All wounds are closed in multiple layers using absorbable suture after copious reirrigation with an antibiotic solution (bacitracin and gentamicin). The device is deactivated and remains deactivated for 6 weeks after surgery (**Fig. 5**). The authors do not routinely place a Foley catheter, allowing the patient to trial void after recovery from anesthesia. If needed, a 12-French Foley catheter is placed in the recovery room and removed 1 to 3 days after surgery. Uncommonly, a percutaneous 12-French supra-pubic catheter is placed at the time of surgery, particularly when a snug cuff fit was used, in which event the urethral catheter may predispose to an early urethral erosion. The patient is discharged the day of surgery with a 7-day course of oral antibiotics and scheduled to return in 6 weeks after surgery for device activation. At that time, a pelvis film is taken before and after activation to ensure adequate transfer of fluid from the pressure-

regulating balloon to the cuff. Patients are seen 3 months after surgery then yearly for review.

REVISIONS

Despite the high success rate and high patient satisfaction after AUS implantation, revision surgery frequently is required for device malfunction, waning continence, and, less commonly, device erosion and infection. After reviewing 119 patients who underwent 159 revision surgeries at the authors' facility, the authors found outcomes for secondary revisions that were comparable with outcomes for primary AUS implantations.[4] Salvage of a good outcome is always possible, even after multiple previous revisions and cuff erosion. Urethral atrophy was the most common cause for device revision and has a number of alternative management options.

In the authors' experience, revision of a device that is not infected or eroded may be done simply and rapidly. Implantation of new device components (pump, balloon, sphincter) into the same pseudocapsule as the old device is safe and results in less morbidity than implantation into a completely new tissue plane. This approach results in minimal postoperative edema and swelling, allowing rapid reactivation of the device and quick return to baseline. The authors have not found any greater incidence of infection with this technique when compared with primary implantation.[4]

Progressively worsening incontinence with a functional device (normal pumping characteristics) implies fluid loss from the system or atrophy of the urethra at the cuff site. The initial evaluation should include a physical examination, pelvis

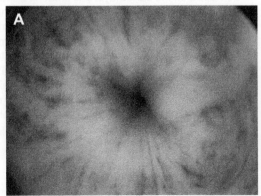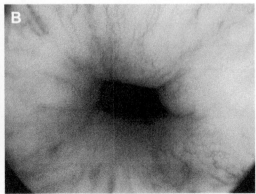

Fig. 4. (*A*) When the AUS is in the closed position, urethroscopy should show slight blanching, indicating adequate coaptation of the device for continence. Under direct endoscopic vision, the cuff is cycled to verify an adequate urethral caliber through which voiding is allowed. (*B*) There should be slight compression of the urethra when the cuff is opened.

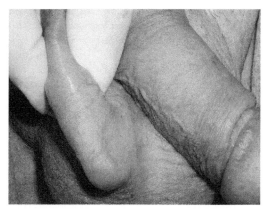

Fig. 5. Deactivation of the device should leave a slight dimple in the control pump that is visible through the scrotal skin.

radiograph, and urethroscopy. Radiographically, increased fluid within the urethral cuff and decreased diameter of the pressure-regulating balloon suggest subcuff atrophy. Urethroscopy should be performed to rule out erosion and often reveals a noncoapted urethra at the cuff site. In the absence of infection and erosion, most cuffs may be downsized in the original location. When a cuff of minimum size (4.0 cm) already has been placed, placement of a tandem cuff, as described by Brito colleagues,[5] may add the extra compression that is needed to obtain continence. The authors prefer to perform revisions in difficult cases with the newly described transcorporal cuff placement.[6]

Transcorporal placement of the AUS provides a number of advantages in difficult cases in which other conventional cuff implantation sites have been used. The corporal tissue included in the cuff dissection potentially protects against a dorsal erosion and allows for cuff placement at a site that would otherwise be too small for even a 4.0-cm cuff. This technique has been described in print and video elsewhere.[6]

AMS expects an average 7- to 10-year life expectancy for most AUSs. For revisions, the authors selected a 3-year cutoff, at which time the entire device is replaced. In the absence of infection or erosion, it is reasonable to replace only the malfunctioning component when revision surgery is performed before 3 years.

A significant improvement in AUS placement is the development of quick connect devices for tubing. Although these devices provide excellent, secure, and watertight connections for newly implanted devices, they cannot be used for revision surgeries. The tubing that is left in place obtains a biofilm, which interferes with the watertight connection. Use of the quick connect devices

results in fluid loss and malfunction. In revision cases in which the entire device is not replaced, tie connectors should be used.

SUMMARY

In correctly chosen and evaluated patients, the AMS model 800 AUS provides excellent long-term outcomes and patient satisfaction. Through years of experience with more than 600 AUS implantations and more than 150 revision surgeries, the authors have developed a quick placement procedure that has minimal complications. Attention to detail is imperative with this surgery, and following the guidelines as listed earlier minimizes postoperative morbidity and complications.

The safe implantation technique as detailed earlier stresses operative field preparation, correct component placement, careful urethral dissection posterior to the crus, and accurate sizing for optimum cuff fit.

ANECDOTAL LESSONS LEARNED AND UNSUBSTANTIATED BELIEFS

1. A patient with a successful AUS placement is the most grateful patient one could wish for.
2. Cuff sizing is the most critical factor in a continent outcome. A higher balloon pressure is not a corrective alternative.
3. Patient expectations may exceed what can be delivered. A patient should not be promised a pad-free future, because going from a 24-hour pad loss weighing 500 mL to one pad a day is success.
4. A significant number of early erosions are caused by urethral compromise at the initial surgery. The authors' technique minimizes this incidence.
5. Intraoperative urethroscopy facilitates cuff sizing.
6. The authors' successful cases include octogenarians. Age is not necessarily a contraindication to implantation.
7. All patients (except for those requiring postoperative cardiac monitoring or coagulation correction) can undergo surgery in an outpatient setting.
8. Filling the device with contrast facilitates follow-up of problems. It allows for easy radiographic diagnosis of device malfunction from system leak and helps identify subcuff urethral atrophy.
9. Other than device leak, subcuff atrophy that results in an oversized cuff is the most common cause for late waning continence. If possible, the cuff can be downsized at the

same site. If a 4-cm cuff was used, a new cuff location (perhaps a proximal relocation or a more distal transcorporal approach) may be required for reimplantation.

10. Revision of the AUS and reoperative surgery result in good outcomes that are on par with outcomes for original implantations.

11. Previous radiation therapy seems to have no significant detrimental effects on good results with AUS implantation.

REFERENCES

1. Elliot DS, Barrett DM. Mayo Clinic long-term analysis of the functional durability of the AMS 800 artificial urinary sphincter: a review of 323 cases. J Urol 1998;159:1206–8.

2. Venn SN, Greenwell TJ, Mundy AR. The long-term outcome of artificial urinary sphincters. J Urol 2000; 164:702–7.

3. Scott EL, Kim KP, Fone PD, et al. Post-prostatectomy incontinence and the artificial urinary sphincter: a long-term study of patient satisfaction and criteria for success. J Urol 2001;156:1975–80.

4. Raj GV, Peterson AC, Toh KL, et al. Outcomes following revision and secondary implantation of the artificial urinary sphincter in cases of device malfunction, urethral atrophy and erosion. J Urol 2003;169(4):19.

5. Brito CG, Mulcahy JJ, Mitchell ME, et al. Use of a double cuff AMS800 urinary sphincter for severe stress incontinence. J Urol 1993;149:283–5.

6. Guralnick ML, Miller EA, Toh KL, et al. Transcorporal artificial urinary sphincter (AUS) cuff placement in cases requiring revision for erosion and urethral atrophy. J Urol 2002;167:2075–9.

Index

Moving?

Make sure your subscription moves with you!

To notify us of your new address, find your **Clinics Account Number** (located on your mailing label above your name), and contact customer service at:

Email: journalscustomerservice-usa@elsevier.com

800-654-2452 (subscribers in the U.S. & Canada)
314-447-8871 (subscribers outside of the U.S. & Canada)

Fax number: 314-447-8029

Elsevier Health Sciences Division
Subscription Customer Service
3251 Riverport Lane
Maryland Heights, MO 63043

*To ensure uninterrupted delivery of your subscription, please notify us at least 4 weeks in advance of move.

Printed and bound by CPI Group (UK) Ltd, Croydon, CR0 4YY

03/10/2024

01040354-0010